Optimal Care for Patients with Epilepsy: Practical Aspects

Editor

STEVEN C. SCHACHTER

NEUROLOGIC CLINICS

www.neurologic.theclinics.com

Consulting Editor
RANDOLPH W. EVANS

May 2016 • Volume 34 • Number 2

ELSEVIER

1600 John F. Kennedy Boulevard • Suite 1800 • Philadelphia, Pennsylvania, 19103-2899

http://www.theclinics.com

NEUROLOGIC CLINICS Volume 34, Number 2
May 2016 ISSN 0733-8619, ISBN-13: 978-0-323-44475-0

Editor: Lauren Boyle
Developmental editor: Donald Mumford

Neurologic Clinics (ISSN 0733-8619) is published quarterly by Elsevier Inc., 360 Park Avenue South, New York, NY 10010–1710. Months of issue are February, May, August, and November. Periodicals postage paid at New York, NY, and additional mailing offices. Subscription prices are $300.00 per year for US individuals, $578.00 per year for US institutions, $100.00 per year for US students, $375.00 per year for Canadian individuals, $701.00 per year for Canadian institutions, $415.00 per year for international individuals, $701.00 per year for international institutions, and $210.00 for Canadian and foreign students/residents. To receive student/resident rate, orders must be accompanied by name of affiliated institution, date of term, and the *signature* of program/residency coordinator on institution letterhead. Orders will be billed at individual rate until proof of status is received. Foreign air speed delivery is included in all *Clinics* subscription prices. All prices are subject to change without notice. **POSTMASTER:** Send address changes to *Neurologic Clinics*, Elsevier Health Sciences Division, Subscription Customer Service, 3251 Riverport Lane, Maryland Heights, MO 63043. **Customer Service: Telephone: 1-800-654-2452 (U.S. and Canada); 314-447-8871 (outside U.S. and Canada). Fax: 314-447-8029. E-mail: journalscustomerservice-usa@elsevier.com (for print support); journalsonlinesupport-usa@elsevier.com (for online support).**

Reprints. For copies of 100 or more of articles in this publication, please contact the Commercial Reprints Department, Elsevier Inc., 360 Park Avenue South, New York, New York, 10010-1710; Tel.: +1-212-633-3874; Fax: +1-212-633-3820, and E-mail: reprints@elsevier.com.

Neurologic Clinics is also published in Spanish by Nueva Editorial Interamericana S.A., Mexico City, Mexico.

Neurologic Clinics is covered in *Current Contents/Clinical Medicine, MEDLINE/PubMed (Index Medicus), EMBASE/Excerpta Medica, and PsycINFO, and ISI/BIOMED.*

Contributors

CONSULTING EDITOR

RANDOLPH W. EVANS, MD
Clinical Professor, Department of Neurology, Baylor College of Medicine, Houston, Texas

EDITOR

STEVEN C. SCHACHTER, MD
Professor of Neurology, Harvard Medical School; Chief Academic Officer, Consortia for Improving Medicine with Innovation and Technology, Boston, Massachusetts

AUTHORS

ANAHITA AGHAEI-LASBOO, MD
Senior Epilepsy Fellow, Department of Neurology and Neurological Sciences, Stanford University School of Medicine, Stanford, California

BENJAMIN N. BLOND, MD
Department of Neurology, Comprehensive Epilepsy Center, Yale University, New Haven, Connecticut

JEFFREY BUCHHALTER, MD, PhD
Professor of Pediatrics and Clinical Neuroscience, Cummings School of Medicine, University of Calgary; Director, Comprehensive Children's Epilepsy Centre, Alberta Children's Hospital, Alberta, Canada

KAMIL DETYNIECKI, MD
Department of Neurology, Comprehensive Epilepsy Center, Yale University, New Haven, Connecticut

COLIN DUNKLEY, MBChB, BSc, MRCPCH
Consultant Paediatrician, Department of Paediatrics, Sherwood Forest Hospitals, Nottinghamshire, United Kingdom

KIRSTEN M. FIEST, PhD
Postdoctoral Fellow, Department of Internal Medicine, Health Sciences Centre, College of Medicine, University of Manitoba, Winnipeg, Manitoba, Canada

ROBERT S. FISHER, MD, PhD
Maslah Saul MD Professor of Neurology, Director Stanford Epilepsy Center, Department of Neurology and Neurological Sciences, Stanford University School of Medicine, Stanford, California

LAWRENCE J. HIRSCH, MD
Department of Neurology, Comprehensive Epilepsy Center, Yale University, New Haven, Connecticut

JENNIFER L. HOPP, MD
Associate Professor, Department of Neurology; Acting Director, Maryland Epilepsy Center, University of Maryland Medical Center, University of Maryland School of Medicine, Baltimore, Maryland

NATHALIE JETTÉ, MD, MSc, FRCPC
Professor, Department of Clinical Neurosciences, Hotchkiss Brain Institute; Department of Community Health Sciences, O'Brien Institute for Public Health, Foothills Medical Centre, Cumming School of Medicine, University of Calgary, Calgary, Alberta, Canada

MARTIN KIRKPATRICK, MBBS, FRCPCH, DCH
Consultant Paediatric Neurologist and Honorary Reader, Department of Child Health, University of Dundee, Dundee, United Kingdom

ALLAN KRUMHOLZ, MD
Professor, Department of Neurology; Director, US Department of Veterans Affairs, Maryland Healthcare System, Epilepsy Center of Excellence, University of Maryland Medical Center, University of Maryland School of Medicine, Baltimore, Maryland

KATHARINE K. McMILLAN, PhD
Research Associate, VA Epilepsy Centers of Excellence, South Texas Veterans Health Care System; Department of Epidemiology and Biostatistics, University of Texas Health Science Center, San Antonio, Texas

SCOTT B. PATTEN, MD, PhD, FRCPC
Professor, Departments of Community Health Sciences, O'Brien Institute for Public Health and Psychiatry, Mathison Centre for Mental Health Research & Education, Foothills Medical Centre, Cumming School of Medicine, University of Calgary, Calgary, Alberta, Canada

PAGE B. PENNELL, MD
Division of Epilepsy, Department of Neurology, Brigham and Women's Hospital, Harvard Medical School, Harvard University; Division of Women's Health, Brigham and Women's Hospital, Harvard Medical School, Harvard University, Boston, Massachusetts

MARY JO PUGH, PhD, RN
Research Scientist, VA Epilepsy Centers of Excellence, South Texas Veterans Health Care System; Associate Professor, Department of Epidemiology and Biostatistics, University of Texas Health Science Center, San Antonio, Texas

ANA M. SANCHEZ, MD
Assistant Professor, Department of Neurology, University of Maryland School of Medicine, Baltimore, Maryland

DIETER SCHMIDT, MD
Emeritus Professor of Neurology; Head, Epilepsy Research Group, Berlin, Germany

PATRICIA OSBORNE SHAFER, RN, MN
Epilepsy Nurse Specialist, Beth Israel Deaconess Medical Center, Boston, Massachusetts; Associate Editor and Community Manager, Epilepsy Foundation, Landover, Maryland

NAYMEÉ J. VÉLEZ-RUIZ, MD
Division of Epilepsy, Department of Neurology, University of Miami, Miami, Florida

SAMUEL WIEBE, MD, MSc, FRCPC
Professor, Department of Clinical Neurosciences, Hotchkiss Brain Institute; Department of Community Health Sciences, O'Brien Institute for Public Health, Foothills Medical Centre, Cumming School of Medicine, University of Calgary, Calgary, Alberta, Canada

Contents

Preface: Practical Approaches to Providing Optimal Care to Patients with Epilepsy   xi

Steven C. Schachter

Guidelines and Quality Standards for Adults with Epilepsy   313

Mary Jo Pugh and Katharine K. McMillan

> Guidelines and quality measures for epilepsy care have the potential to improve the quality of epilepsy care. Quality measures are increasingly used for pay-for-performance. This article describes different guidelines and quality measures that have been used to identify best practices, types of best practices for use in clinical care developed using each of these approaches, and information on how to interpret the recommendations in specific guidelines and quality measures described elsewhere in this issue.

Guidelines and Quality Standards in the Care of Children with Epilepsy   327

Martin Kirkpatrick and Colin Dunkley

> To provide quality care for children with epilepsy there is a continuing need to synthesize clinical research into forms that reflect best clinical practice. The design of evidence-based guidelines allows the gathering of this information together. This review discusses the components needed to analyze published data and produce recommendations for clinical management. Guideline implementation should be seen as an essential component that is integrated into guideline development. Robust clinical practice guidelines can also form the basis of defining quality standards that in turn should allow the development and measurement of clinical outcomes that lead to direct improvements in patient care.

Initial Evaluation of the Patient with Suspected Epilepsy   339

Nathalie Jetté and Samuel Wiebe

> The initial evaluation of the patient with suspected epilepsy is multifaceted and includes a careful history, diagnostic evaluation (EEG and brain imaging) and prompt referral to an epilepsy specialist to clarify seizure types and epilepsy syndrome. Screening for mental health conditions also should be considered, along with neurocognitive testing when deficits of language, memory, learning, attention, or executive function are present or when MRI shows involvement of brain regions implicated in cognitive function. In this review, we examine the approach to the initial evaluation of those with new-onset unprovoked seizures and possible epilepsy.

Screening for Depression and Anxiety in Epilepsy   351

Kirsten M. Fiest, Scott B. Patten, and Nathalie Jetté

> Depression and anxiety are common comorbidities of epilepsy and have far-reaching effects on patients, family, and the health care system.

Although the burden of these conditions is high, a majority of cases are undetected and untreated. Screening tools can be a fast way to establish the presence of clinically relevant symptoms of depression and anxiety in epilepsy. Depression tools have been extensively studied in epilepsy, although no scale has been definitively established for use in this population. Anxiety has been understudied in epilepsy; few scales exist to measure anxiety and these scales have not been well validated.

Starting, Choosing, Changing, and Discontinuing Drug Treatment for Epilepsy Patients   363

Dieter Schmidt

Epilepsy is a serious brain disease with seizures as the main symptom, which can be successfully treated with antiepileptic drugs (AEDs). AEDs are usually started as soon as the epilepsy diagnosis has been established. About 80% of adults with new-onset epilepsy will achieve lasting seizure remission on AEDs. However, 20% continue to have seizures despite treatment (drug-resistant epilepsy). AEDs can be safely discontinued after several years of seizure remission during early treatment. Remarkably, 60% of all treated patients remain in remission off AEDs, making epilepsy one of the best treatable among chronic brain diseases.

Methods for Measuring Seizure Frequency and Severity   383

Anahita Aghaei-Lasboo and Robert S. Fisher

Counting seizures is not simple. Patients may not be aware of their seizures. Adherence to diary entry often is poor. Shake detectors pick up only seizures with rhythmic movements and suffer from false-positive results. Measurement of electrodermal response is a promising technology but sensitivity and specificity for partial seizures are uncertain. Video-electroencephalogram monitoring is accurate but of short duration and performed in an artificial and expensive environment. Invasive electroencephalogram electrodes can detect seizure-like patterns, sometimes of unknown clinical significance. Practical long-term electroencephalogram monitors are under development. Methods to rank seizure severity are subjective. New approaches and solutions are needed.

Assessment of Treatment Side Effects and Quality of Life in People with Epilepsy   395

Benjamin N. Blond, Kamil Detyniecki, and Lawrence J. Hirsch

Epilepsy impairs quality of life in physical, psychological, cognitive, social, and occupational domains. In people who are not seizure free, depression and adverse medication effects have a predominant role in determining quality of life. The assessment of these factors and other comorbidities is essential for maximizing quality of life in epilepsy. There are multiple tools available to assess medication effects and quality of life in a structured format. Such tools can provide superior assessments and allow clinicians to have a greater impact on their patients' quality of life.

Issues for Women with Epilepsy   **411**

Naymeé J. Vélez-Ruiz and Page B. Pennell

Epilepsy and antiepileptic drugs affect the menstrual cycle, aspects of contraception, reproductive health, pregnancy, and menopause through alteration of sex steroid hormone pathways. Sex steroid hormones often have an effect on seizure frequency and may alter the level of some antiepileptic drugs. Approximately one-third of women experience an increase in perimenstrual and/or periovulatory seizure frequency. Some women experience an increase in seizure frequency during pregnancy. Balancing maternal seizure control and the risk of congenital malformations associated with fetal antiepileptic drug exposure may be challenging. Some antiepileptic drugs are associated with cognitive and behavioral teratogenesis and should be avoided if possible during pregnancy.

Counseling Epilepsy Patients on Driving and Employment   **427**

Allan Krumholz, Jennifer L. Hopp, and Ana M. Sanchez

People with epilepsy identify driving and employment among their major concerns. People with controlled seizures may be permitted to drive in every state in the United States, but people with uncontrolled seizures are restricted from licensure. Unemployment and underemployment for people with epilepsy are serious problems that depend on the frequency and type of seizure disorder and associated medical and psychological problems. Most jobs, with reasonable accommodation by employers, are suitable for people with epilepsy. Federal protections through the Americans with Disabilities Act confer civil rights protection by law on people with disabilities such as epilepsy.

Patient Education: Identifying Risks and Self-Management Approaches for Adherence and Sudden Unexpected Death in Epilepsy   **443**

Patricia Osborne Shafer and Jeffrey Buchhalter

Patient education in epilepsy is one part of quality epilepsy care and is an evolving and growing field. Health outcomes, patient satisfaction, safety, patient/provider communication, and quality of life may all be affected by what people are taught (or not taught), what they understand, and how they use this information to make decisions and manage their health. Data regarding learning needs and interventions to address medication adherence and sudden unexpected death in epilepsy education can be used to guide clinicians in health care or community settings.

Index   **457**

FORTHCOMING ISSUES

August 2016
Case Studies in Neurology
Randolph Evans, *Editor*

November 2016
Global and Domestic Public Health and Neuroepidemiology
David Younger, *Editor*

February 2017
Neuro-Ophthalmology
Andrew Lee, *Editor*

RECENT ISSUES

February 2016
Neurobehavioral Manifestations of Neurological Diseases: Diagnosis and Treatment
Alireza Minagar, Glen Finney, and Kenneth M. Heilman, *Editors*

November 2015
Motor Neuron Disease
Richard J. Barohn and Mazen Dimachkie, *Editors*

August 2015
Emergency Neuro-Otology: Diagnosis and Management of Acute Dizziness and Vertigo
David E. Newman-Toker, Kevin A. Kerber, William J. Meurer, Rodney Omron, and Jonathan A. Edlow, *Editors*

RELATED INTEREST

Neurosurgery Clinics, January 2016 (Vol. 27, Issue 1, p. 1–136)
Epilepsy
Kareem A. Zaghloul and Edward F. Chang, *Editors*

THE CLINICS ARE AVAILABLE ONLINE!
Access your subscription at:
www.theclinics.com

Preface

Practical Approaches to Providing Optimal Care to Patients with Epilepsy

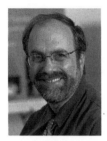

Steven C. Schachter, MD
Editor

The many time, financial, and clinical pressures on busy practicing clinicians make it increasingly challenging to efficiently and consistently provide high-quality care for patients with epilepsy. Further compounding this situation are continually evolving treatment options, diagnostic tests, quality-of-care metrics, guidelines, and clinical decision rules for epilepsy.

This issue of *Neurologic Clinics* addresses this situation through a series of articles written by renowned experts. First, quality standards, practice guidelines, and related consensus statements for the care of adults and children with epilepsy are reviewed. Second, methods for their application to clinical practice using validated and evidence-based tools such as screening instruments and algorithms are presented in the context of critically important topics that arise in daily clinical practice.

Steven C. Schachter, MD
Harvard Medical School
Consortia for Improving Medicine
with Innovation & Technology 125 Nashua Street
Suite 3228
Boston, MA 02114, USA

E-mail address:
sschacht@bidmc.harvard.edu

Neurol Clin 34 (2016) xi
http://dx.doi.org/10.1016/j.ncl.2016.02.001
0733-8619/16/$ – see front matter © 2016 Published by Elsevier Inc.

neurologic.theclinics.com

Guidelines and Quality Standards for Adults with Epilepsy

Mary Jo Pugh, PhD, RN[a,b,*], Katharine K. McMillan, PhD[a,b]

KEYWORDS

- Epilepsy • Guidelines • Quality measures • Quality indicators
- Evidence-based practice

KEY POINTS

- Definitions of high-quality care exist in the form of guidelines and quality measures.
- Guidelines include focused evidence-based guidelines that address specific clinical issues, such as care for women with epilepsy, and clinical practice guidelines that address comprehensive disease management.
- Quality indicators identify specific processes of care that are tightly linked to patient outcomes.
- Guidelines and quality indicators can be used to guide clinical judgment and improve quality of epilepsy care.

Since the 1970s there has been increasing interest in improving the quality of care provided to patients by leveraging information from the vast and growing body of biomedical research. This interest resulted in developing approaches to compile the existing evidence and develop evidence-based recommendations for care in the form of clinical practice guidelines (CPGs) and later, quality measures to improve the quality of health care.

Disclosure Statement: The authors have nothing to disclose.
VA Health Services Research and Development (IIR 11-067; Dr M.J. Pugh PI) funded this study. The content of this article is solely the responsibility of the authors and does not necessarily reflect the official views of the Veterans' Health Administration. The funding organizations had no role in the design and conduct of the study; the collection, management, analysis, and interpretation of the data; or the preparation, review, or approval of the article.
[a] South Texas Veterans Health Care System (11C6), 7400 Merton Minter Boulevard, San Antonio, TX 78229, USA; [b] Department of Epidemiology and Biostatistics, 7703 Floyd Curl Drive, San Antonio, TX 78229, USA
* Corresponding author. South Texas Veterans Health Care System (11C6), 7400 Merton Minter Boulevard, San Antonio, TX 78229.
E-mail addresses: MaryJoPugh2@va.gov; pughm@uthscsa.edu

Neurol Clin 34 (2016) 313–325
http://dx.doi.org/10.1016/j.ncl.2015.11.006
0733-8619/16/$ – see front matter Published by Elsevier Inc.
neurologic.theclinics.com

Although the definitions of quality have changed over time, there is growing consensus around the definition put forth by the Agency for Healthcare Research and Quality: providing the right care to the right patient at the right time and in the right way to achieve the best possible results.[1] The foundation of this definition is the identification of what is the right care. Accordingly, much work has been done to identify these "best practices" over the past 30 years. Identification of best practices began more recently for epilepsy, so clinicians may be less familiar with this process. This article describes different guidelines and quality measures that have been used to identify best practices, types of best practices for use in clinical care developed using each of these approaches, and information on how to interpret the recommendations in specific guidelines and quality measures that are described elsewhere in this issue.

GUIDELINES FOR CLINICAL CARE

Review of the literature for epilepsy guidelines revealed two general types. The first is an evidence-based practice parameter/guideline that addresses a single clinical focus and that results in recommendations based on the synthesis of evidence available in the literature. The second is a comprehensive disease CPG.

Clinically Focused Guidelines

Single-focus guidelines are generally developed by a professional society, such as the American Academy of Neurology (AAN), the American Epilepsy Society, or the International League Against Epilepsy (ILAE). This process begins with a clinical question of interest identified by members of the professional society. Next, a panel of experts is convened as a scientific team to conduct a rigorous systematic review of the available evidence. This process begins with a broad search of the literature, based on a priori inclusion and exclusion criteria. For instance, the evaluation of management of a first unprovoked seizure in adults included randomized controlled trials, case-control or cohort studies, and case series with 10 or more participants.[2] It further restricted its literature search to first seizure reporting in individuals 18 years and older. Articles that examined children (<18 years), review articles, meta-analyses, and small case series studies (<10 individuals) were excluded.

Once articles that meet inclusion criteria are identified, the team reviews titles and abstracts to ensure that all studies meet inclusion criteria. Relevant papers are then classified a priori based on study design and then undergo full-text review to identify evidence that addresses specific clinical questions. The classification and evaluation scheme for grading the quality of evidence follows strict guidelines established by the organization.[3,4] The scientific team compiles recommendations, and the strength of each recommendation is classified based on the level of supporting evidence in the literature. The benefit of this rigorous, systematic process is that clinicians can access this concise review of the literature, examine these evidence-based recommendations, and determine a course of action for patient care based on patient characteristics and the level of evidence for specific recommendations. However, classification systems for understanding the strength of recommendations are complex.[5]

Table 1 provides a description of the level of recommendations used in AAN practice parameters/guidelines (terminology in descriptors changed over time; hereafter we use guidelines).[6] The clearest recommendations are Level A, which identifies processes of care or diagnostic approaches that have established efficacy, harm, or lack of efficacy based on the literature; and U, which identifies processes of care or diagnostic approaches that lack adequate data to make a determination. **Table 1** also identifies the types of studies that are required to meet specific evidence levels. Thus, these guidelines are not entirely prescriptive, but rather provide clinicians with a concise summary of the literature that can be used to inform clinical decisions.[7]

This process has been used by professional societies to develop a large number of focused, evidence-based guidelines for specific areas of clinical care, which are updated as new evidence becomes available. **Table 2** provides some examples of existing (AAN, ILAE) focused, evidence-based guidelines that can be accessed on the Internet and the World Wide Web link for each guideline. Guidelines exist for a variety of issues related to pharmacologic treatment of new-onset epilepsy,[8–10] refractory epilepsy,[11] patients with human immunodeficiency virus/AIDS,[12] women's health issues,[13–15] and other topics.[16–19] In addition, the AAN is currently developing guidelines regarding sudden unexplained death in epilepsy and timing of antiepileptic drug withdrawal in seizure-free patients with epilepsy. Guidelines and resources for clinicians and patients are available at www.aan.com/Guidelines and www.ilae.org.

Comprehensive Guidelines

In addition to clinically focused guidelines, comprehensive disease-focused CPGs have been developed in the United Kingdom and other countries, although none were developed in the United States. Like the clinically focused guidelines, the process of CPG development is based on a systematic review of the literature, synthesis of that evidence to form recommendations with a description of the strength of the evidence, and external review to ensure accuracy of the information. AAN,[20] National Institute for Health and Care Excellence (NICE),[21] and ILAE[22] provide opportunities for public comment before publication of their respective approved guidelines. The Scottish Intercollegiate Guideline Network (SIGN) submits their guidelines to a peer-review process of reviewers selected by the organization.[23,24] However, unlike clinically focused guidelines, additional sources of evidence including expert opinion may be used as evidence. Randomized control trials for some processes of care are not practical or are unethical to conduct. For instance it is important for patients to know the side-effects of medications and to understand their disease process if they are to be proactive informed partners in caring for their chronic disease.[3] Moreover, clinicians know the critical importance of informing patients with epilepsy about potential risks for injury including driving restrictions, yet clinical trials have not been done to demonstrate the efficacy of these care processes. Therefore expert opinion is an important component of guideline development, and clinicians are able to clearly identify those clinical recommendations that are based on expert opinion.

Table 3 provides information for two CPGs that address care for adults with epilepsy, one of which was developed by SIGN, and the other developed by NICE in the United Kingdom early in the 2000s and that have been recently updated based on new evidence. The NICE guideline addresses care for children and adults,[21] and the SIGN 143[25] focuses exclusively on care for adults. Both SIGN 143 and NICE guidelines are targeted for primary care and secondary care and address diagnosis, pharmacologic treatment, nondrug treatment and adjunctive therapy, women's health issues, and special needs for older people (65+) with epilepsy. Although many of these topics are addressed from the perspective of US clinicians in the professional society focused guidelines, topics include issues of design of epilepsy care and models of epilepsy care that are not directly relevant to the system of care in the

Table 1
Defining levels of recommendation used in American Academy of Neurology evidence-based guidelines

Level of Recommendation	Evidence Required for Recommendation	Classification of Evidence
A = Established as effective, ineffective, or harmful (or established as useful/predictive or not useful/predictive) for the given condition in the specified population	Requires at least two consistent Class I studies[a]	Class I: A randomized, controlled clinical trial of the intervention of interest with masked or objective outcome assessment, in a representative population. Relevant baseline characteristics are presented and substantially equivalent among treatment groups or there is appropriate statistical adjustment for differences. The following are also required: a. Concealed allocation b. Primary outcomes clearly defined c. Exclusion/inclusion criteria clearly defined d. Adequate accounting for dropouts (with at least 80% of enrolled subjects completing the study) and crossovers with numbers sufficiently low to have minimal potential for bias e. For noninferiority or equivalence trials claiming to prove efficacy for one or both drugs, the following are also required[a]: i. The authors explicitly state the clinically meaningful difference to be excluded by defining the threshold for equivalence or noninferiority ii. The standard treatment used in the study is substantially similar to that used in previous studies establishing efficacy of the standard treatment (eg, for a drug, the mode of administration, dose, and dosage adjustments are similar to those previously shown to be effective) iii. The inclusion and exclusion criteria for patient selection and the outcomes of patients on the standard treatment are comparable with those of previous studies establishing efficacy of the standard treatment iv. The interpretation of the results of the study is based on a per-protocol analysis that takes into account dropouts or crossovers

B = Probably effective, ineffective, or harmful (or probably useful/predictive or not useful/predictive) for the given condition in the specified population	Requires at least one Class I study or two consistent Class II studies	Class II: A randomized, controlled clinical trial of the intervention of interest in a representative population with masked or objective outcome assessment that lacks one criteria a–e above or a prospective matched cohort study with masked or objective outcome assessment in a representative population that meets b–e above. Relevant baseline characteristics are presented and substantially equivalent among treatment groups or there is appropriate statistical adjustment for differences.
C = Possibly effective, ineffective, or harmful (or possibly useful/predictive or not useful/predictive) for the given condition in the specified population	Requires at least one Class II study or two consistent Class III studies	Class III: All other controlled trials (including well-defined natural history control subjects or patients serving as own control subjects) in a representative population, where outcome is independently assessed, or independently derived by objective outcome measurement.[b]
U = Data inadequate or conflicting; given current knowledge, treatment (test, predictor) is unproven	Assigned in cases of only one Class III study, only Class IV studies, or evidence that is conflicting and cannot be reconciled	Class IV: Studies not meeting Class I, II, or III criteria, including consensus or expert opinion.

Notes: Recommendations can be positive or negative.
[a] Note that numbers i–iii in Class I, item e, are required for Class II in equivalence trials. If any one of the three is missing, the class is automatically downgraded to Class III.
[b] Objective outcome measurement: an outcome measure that is unlikely to be affected by an observer's (patient, treating physician, investigator) expectation or bias (eg, blood tests, administrative outcome data).
From Evidence-based Guideline for Clinicians: Management of an Unprovoked First Seizure in Adults [presentation slides]. Minneapolis, MN: American Academy of Neurology; April 21, 2015. https://www.aan.com/Guidelines/Home/GetGuidelineContent/690. Slides 17-20. Accessed: July 4, 2015. Used by permission.

Table 2
Examples of clinically focused evidence-based guidelines

Guideline	Developer	Year (Prior Versions)
Management of an unprovoked first seizure in adults http://www.neurology.org/content/84/16/1705.full	AAN AES	2015
Vagus nerve stimulation for the treatment of epilepsy http://www.neurology.org/content/81/16/1453.full	AAN	2013
Treatment of parenchymal neurocysticercosis http://www.neurology.org/content/80/15/1424.full	AAN	2003
Antiepileptic drug selection for people with human immunodeficiency virus/AIDS http://www.neurology.org/content/78/2/139.full.html	AAN ILAE	2012
Efficacy and tolerability of the new antiepileptic drugs I: treatment of new-onset epilepsy http://www.neurology.org/content/62/8/1252.full	AAN AES	2004 (currently under review)
Efficacy and tolerability of the new antiepileptic drugs II: treatment of refractory epilepsy http://www.neurology.org/content/62/8/1261.full	AAN AES	2004 (currently under review)
Temporal lobe and localized neocortical resections for epilepsy http://www.neurology.org/content/60/4/538.full	AAN AES AANS	2008 (2003, 2005)
Practice advisory: the use of felbamate in the treatment of patients with intractable epilepsy http://www.neurology.org/content/52/8/1540.full	AAN AES	2013 (1999, 2003, 2006, 2010)
Updated ILAE evidence review of antiepileptic drug efficacy and effectiveness as initial monotherapy for epileptic seizures and syndromes http://www.ilae.org/Visitors/Documents/Guidelines-epilepsia-12074-2013.pdf	ILAE	2013
ILAE treatment guidelines: evidence-based analysis of antiepileptic drug efficacy and effectiveness as initial monotherapy for epileptic seizures and syndromes http://www.ilae.org/visitors/Documents/Guidelines.pdf	ILAE	2006
Practice parameter update: management issues for women with epilepsy—focus on pregnancy (an evidence-based review): obstetric complications and change in seizure frequency http://www.neurology.org/content/73/2/126.full.html	AAN	2013 (2009)
Practice parameter update: management issues for women with epilepsy—focus on pregnancy (an evidence-based review): teratogenesis and perinatal outcomes http://www.neurology.org/content/73/2/133.full.html	AAN	2013 (2009)
Update: management issues for women with epilepsy-focus on pregnancy: vitamin K, folic acid, blood levels, and breastfeeding http://www.neurology.org/content/73/2/142.full.html	AAN	2013 (2009)

Note: AAN guidelines for epilepsy and clinician and patient resources can be found at https://www.aan.com/Guidelines/Home/ByTopic?topicId=23. More updates and guideline information can be found at International League Against Epilepsy, http://www.ilae.org/Visitors/Centre/Guidelines.cfm.
Abbreviations: AANS, American Academy of Neurosurgeons; AES, American Epilepsy Society.

Table 3 Broad disease-based guidelines		
Guideline	**Developer**	**Year (Prior Versions)**
The epilepsies: the diagnosis and management of the epilepsies in adults and children in primary and secondary care. (Guideline 137) www.nice.org.uk/guidance/cg137	National Institute for Health and Care Excellence	2012 (2004)
Diagnosis and management of epilepsy in adults (Guideline 143) www.sign.ac.uk	Scottish Intercollegiate Guidelines Network	2015 (SIGN 70, 2003)

United States; however, these recommendations may be examined by US clinicians to determine feasibility in our different system of care.

QUALITY INDICATORS AND QUALITY MEASURES

The purpose of guidelines is to identify best practices for clinical care, but quality indicators (QIs) and quality measurement were developed as a tool for quality improvement and more recently for accountability.[26] As such, the development of QIs is different than guidelines because not only is it important to identify processes of care that are appropriate in specific settings, but it is also important to identify processes of care that are feasible to measure and tightly linked to patient outcomes. Like guidelines, QI development begins with a systematic review of the literature to identify best practices. Evidence syntheses, such as AAN guidelines and comprehensive CPGs, often provide the foundation for quality measure development.[27] Unlike guidelines, however, QIs typically use an expert consensus process to review the evidence supporting each QI and rate the feasibility of measurement.[28]

Although quality measure development began late for epilepsy compared with other chronic diseases, the implications for quality measurement in the current clinical climate are the same for all health conditions.[29] In the past, the focus of quality measurement was at the institution and health care system level, where individuals within the institution developed programs to measure and improve the quality of care. More recently, external quality assurance models, such as the Medicare Hospital Compare program, improved transparency of hospital quality by providing data from Medicare-certified acute care hospitals that allowed consumers to compare the quality of care at different hospitals. Current metrics include time to access care, complications after surgery, hospital readmissions, patient satisfaction, and other important measures.[30] In the last decade quality measurement has been used for accountability of clinicians and institutions in "pay-for-performance" programs where a small financial incentive was provided to encourage reporting of quality of care.[31] Since 2011, facilities have been required to report results for three epilepsy quality measures to the Centers for Medicare and Medicaid Service (CMS) to avoid a 2% reduction in reimbursement for epilepsy services.[29] Although clinical leaders specializing in other conditions, such as hypertension and diabetes, had more than a decade of quality improvement experience before the pay-for-performance mandates, epilepsy clinicians had little time to understand this system because the AAN quality measures for epilepsy were published in 2011, the same year as mandatory reporting for epilepsy quality measures.[32] Therefore, understanding the development and content of existing epilepsy quality measures is critically important for clinicians.

HISTORY OF EPILEPSY QUALITY MEASURES

The Centers for Disease Control and Prevention identified the need for epilepsy quality measures in the early 2000s and developed two funded programs: one for children and one for adults.[33] The concern that only about half of adults with epilepsy received care from a neurologist in a given year led the Centers for Disease Control and Prevention to focus on QIs for patients seen in primary care.[34] The result of the Quality Indicators in Epilepsy Treatment (QUIET) study was a series of 24 evidence-based QI and five QI that were based on focus groups with patients with epilepsy.[35] Evidence-based QIs, developed by evaluating existing CPGs and systematic review of the literature, included processes of care associated with evaluation of a first seizure, treatment of incident epilepsy, chronic epilepsy care, and issues specific to women. The patient-generated QI focused primarily on psychosocial aspects of epilepsy. Although helpful in guiding primary care clinicians, the number of QIs makes it difficult to provide a comprehensive assessment of epilepsy care quality, and most of the QIs are impossible to measure without medical chart abstraction (a sample QUIET chart abstraction tool may be downloaded from www.epilepsy.va.gov/quiet).

AMERICAN ACADEMY OF NEUROLOGY QUALITY MEASURE SETS
American Academy of Neurology 2009 Quality Measure Set

The AAN used the QUIET indicators[35,36] as a foundation for QI development, identifying specific processes of care for which there was thought to be a gap in the quality of care, there was high-quality evidence, and strongly associated with patient outcomes.[32] Using the process outlined by the Physician Consortium for Performance Improvement of the American Medical Association including systematic review of the literature, eight measures were approved by the multidisciplinary panel.[37] These eight measures of the AAN Quality Measure set (AAN-QM) were then submitted to CMS for approval as pay-for-performance measures. **Table 4** shows the specific measures that were approved and the three QI that were approved as pay-for-performance measures by CMS. Of concern to the AAN Quality Measurement and Reporting Subcommittee was a more recent decision by the National Quality Forum (NQF) to endorse only QI Number 8, focused on providing counseling on issues specific to women, because this may eventually be reflected in pay-for-performance measures as CMS typically only approves quality measures approved by the NQF.[29] In part the lack of endorsement was associated with concern that other AAN-QM items were not tightly linked to patient outcomes.

Research using the original AAN-QM suggests that gaps in epilepsy care exist. Pourdeyhimi and colleagues[38] used medical chart abstraction to evaluate quality of care in a specialty care setting using AAN-QM and found that quality of care was significantly higher for patients receiving epilepsy specialty care than for patients seen in primary care. Moreover, adherence to AAN-QM gradually diminished from initial to follow-up visits, and the presence of ongoing seizures improved AAN-QM concordant care. Another approach to examining the AAN-QM concordant care was introduced by Wicks and Fountain.[39] After developing a survey to measure patient self-reported quality of care, they deployed the survey in an existing online community (Patients Like Me, epilepsy community). The items in the survey identified the extent to which patients reported receiving each of the AAN-QM, and found that individuals receiving neurology and epilepsy specialty care received a higher proportion of care processes than individuals who received only primary care (~87% vs 70%).[39]

Despite the existence of QM for nearly 5 years, published studies examining the association of AAN-QM concordant epilepsy care and patient outcomes have only

Table 4
American Academy of Neurology quality measures

2009 Measure Set	2014 Measure Set
1. Seizure types and current frequencies documented: each encounter[a]	1A. Seizure frequency documented: each visit (2009 measure revised) 1B. Seizure intervention offered or discussed: each encounter where seizure count >0 (2009 measure revised)
2. Etiology of epilepsy or epilepsy syndrome documented: each encounter[a]	2. Etiology, seizure type, and epilepsy syndrome documented OR testing ordered to determine cause, seizure type, epilepsy syndrome: each encounter
3. Electroencephalogram results reviewed, requested, or test ordered: initial evaluation	Retired
4. MRI/computed tomography scan results reviewed, requested, or scan ordered: initial evaluation	Retired
5. Antiepileptic drug side effects evaluated: each encounter	3. Intervention provided for individuals with active side effects from antiseizure therapy: each encounter for those with side effects reported on query
6. Surgical evaluation considered: every 3 y for intractable	Retired
7. Counseling for safety issues: yearly	4. Counseling for personalized safety issues and epilepsy education: yearly
8: Counseling for issues specific to women: yearly for women of childbearing potential (12–44 y)[a,b]	5. Counseling for issues specific to women: yearly for women of childbearing potential (12–44 y); reaffirmed
—	6. Screening for psychiatric or behavioral health disorders documented: each encounter (new measure)
—	7. Referral to comprehensive epilepsy center: every 2 y for patients with treatment-resistant epilepsy (new measure)

[a] Items approved by the Centers for Medicaid and Medicare services for pay for performance.
[b] Items approved by the National Quality Forum as a valid quality measure.

begun to emerge. Ladner and colleagues[40] examined the association between receiving AAN-QM concordant care and epilepsy-related adverse hospitalizations. Findings suggest that epilepsy-related adverse hospitalizations were associated only with documentation of seizure frequency. Pitfalls identified in QM development for other chronic diseases include identifying processes of care that are far removed from patient outcomes, and which may be most important for individuals at highest risk.[41,42] Ladner's finding that documentation of seizure frequency (and possibly associated interventions to address refractory seizures) supports the notion that this particular AAN-QM is tightly associated with the specific outcome measured: epilepsy-related adverse hospitalizations. More research is needed to address outcomes associated with AAN-QM concordant care before clinicians can determine the quality of AAN-QM. However, identification of appropriate outcomes for each measure should first be identified.

American Academy of Neurology 2014 Quality Measure Set

In 2014 the AAN convened a second Epilepsy Measure Development Panel to evaluate the evidence for existing measures and determine if new measures were warranted based on recommendations from the Institute of Medicine Report (*Epilepsy Across the Spectrum: Promoting Health and Understanding*), new evidence, and desirable attributes of performance measures. Based on prior experience with the NQF, the focus of this evaluation involved a special emphasis on the link between specific performance measures and outcomes relevant to patients with epilepsy.[41–43]

Table 4 shows the 2014 AAN-QM items that were approved by the measure development panel alongside the previously approved 2009 AAN-QM items. From the original eight AAN-QM, three items were retired, four measures were revised to reflect new evidence, and the item regarding women of childbearing potential was reaffirmed. In addition, two new items addressing mental health screening and referral to a comprehensive epilepsy center were added. These new measures will also be submitted for consideration to the Physician Quality Reporting System and CMS to identify potentially new pay-for-performance measures.

IMPLEMENTING HIGH-QUALITY CARE IN YOUR PRACTICE

In line with the 2012 Institute of Medicine recommendations for epilepsy care, gaps in care quality must be addressed.[43] To do so, however, it is critical to understand the care that is currently being provided, and identify the gaps in quality. Existing guidelines and quality measures provide definitions of high-quality care that research and quality improvement programs can use to benchmark the quality of care provided using data gathered by electronic health records. The ability to feed the information on gaps observed in quality back to clinicians allows development of a "learning health care system" where data from routine clinical care are eventually used to provide guidance for physicians at the point of care.[44,45] Such a research agenda would address recommendations of the Institute of Medicine to improve the quality of care for patients with epilepsy and develop a national system of quality measurement.[43]

REFERENCES

1. National Committee for Quality Assurance (NCQA). The essential guide to health care quality. Washington, DC: NCQA; 2007.
2. Krumholz A, Wiebe S, Gronseth G, et al. Evidence-based guideline: management of an unprovoked first seizure in adults. Neurology 2015;84:1705–13.
3. French J, Gronseth G. Lost in a jungle of evidence: we need a compass. Neurology 2008;71(20):1634–8.
4. Gronseth G, French J. Practice parameters and technology assessments: what they are, what they are not, and why you should care. Neurology 2008;71(20):1639–43.
5. Lohr KN. Rating the strength of scientific evidence: relevance for quality improvement programs. Int J Qual Health Care 2004;16(1):9–18.
6. American Academy of Neurology. Evidence-based guideline for clinicians: management of an unprovoked first seizure in adults [presentation slides]. Available at: https://www.aan.com/Guidelines/Home/GetGuidelineContent/690. Accessed April 21, 2015.
7. Getchius TS, Moses LK, French J, et al. AAN guidelines: a benefit to the neurologist. Neurology 2010;75(13):1126–7.

8. French JA, Kanner AM, Bautista J, et al. Efficacy and tolerability of the new anti-epileptic drugs I: treatment of new onset epilepsy: report of the therapeutics and technology assessment subcommittee and quality standards subcommittee of the American Academy of Neurology and the American Epilepsy Society. Neurology 2004;62(8):1252–60.

9. Glauser T, Ben-Menachem E, Bourgeois B, et al. ILAE treatment guidelines: evidence-based analysis of antiepileptic drug efficacy and effectiveness as initial monotherapy for epileptic seizures and syndromes. Epilepsia 2006;47(7):1094–120.

10. Glauser T, Ben-Menachem E, Bourgeois B, et al. Updated ILAE evidence review of antiepileptic drug efficacy and effectiveness as initial monotherapy for epileptic seizures and syndromes. Epilepsia 2013;54(3):551–63.

11. French J, Kanner A, Bautista J, et al. Efficacy and tolerability of the new antiepileptic drugs II: treatment of refractory epilepsy: report of the therapeutics and technology assessment subcommittee and quality standards subcommittee of the American Academy of Neurology and the American Epilepsy Society. Neurology 2004;62(8):1261–73.

12. Birbeck GL, French JA, Perucca E, et al. Antiepileptic drug selection for people with HIV/AIDS: evidence-based guidelines from the ILAE and AAN. Epilepsia 2012;53(1):207–14.

13. Harden CL, Hopp J, Ting TY, et al. Practice parameter update: management issues for women with epilepsy–focus on pregnancy (an evidence-based review): obstetrical complications and change in seizure frequency: report of the quality standards subcommittee and therapeutics and technology assessment subcommittee of the American Academy of Neurology and American Epilepsy Society. Neurology 2009;73(2):126–32.

14. Harden CL, Meador KJ, Pennell PB, et al. Practice parameter update: management issues for women with epilepsy–focus on pregnancy (an evidence-based review): teratogenesis and perinatal outcomes: report of the quality standards subcommittee and therapeutics and technology assessment subcommittee of the American Academy of Neurology and American Epilepsy Society. Neurology 2009;73(2):133–41.

15. Harden CL, Pennell PB, Koppel BS, et al. Practice parameter update: management issues for women with epilepsy–focus on pregnancy (an evidence-based review): vitamin K, folic acid, blood levels, and breastfeeding: report of the quality standards subcommittee and therapeutics and technology assessment subcommittee of the American Academy of Neurology and American Epilepsy Society. Neurology 2009;73(2):142–9.

16. Morris GL, Gloss D, Buchhalter J, et al. Evidence-based guideline update: vagus nerve stimulation for the treatment of epilepsy report of the guideline development subcommittee of the American Academy of Neurology. Neurology 2013;81(16):1453–9.

17. Baird RA, Wiebe S, Zunt JR, et al. Evidence-based guideline: treatment of parenchymal neurocysticercosis: report of the Guideline Development Subcommittee of the American Academy of Neurology. Neurology 2013;80(15):1424–9.

18. Engel J Jr, Wiebe S, French J, et al. Practice parameter: temporal lobe and localized neocortical resections for epilepsy: report of the quality standards subcommittee of the American Academy of Neurology, in association with the American Epilepsy Society and the American Association of Neurological Surgeons. Neurology 2003;60(4):538–47.

19. French J, Smith M, Faught E, et al. Practice advisory: the use of felbamate in the treatment of patients with intractable epilepsy: report of the quality standards

subcommittee of the American Academy of Neurology and the American Epilepsy Society. Neurology 1999;52(8):1540–5.

20. Fountain NB, Van Ness PC, Bennett A, et al. Quality improvement in neurology: Epilepsy Update Quality Measurement Set. Neurology 2015;84(14):1483–7.

21. National Institute for Health and Care Excellence (NICE). The epilepsies: the diagnosis and management of the epilepsies in adults and children in primary and secondary care (CG137). London: NICE; 2012.

22. International League Against Epilepsy (ILAE). Guidelines for publications from League commissions and task forces. 2013.

23. Scottish Intercollegiate Guidelines Network, Harbour RT, Forsyth L. SIGN 50: a guideline developer's handbook. Edinburgh (United Kingdom): Scottish Intercollegiate Guidelines Network; 2008.

24. Scottish Intercollegiate Guidelines Network (SIGN). Guideline development in fifty easy steps. Available at: http://www.sign.ac.uk/pdf/50steps.pdf. Accessed July 6, 2015.

25. Scottish Intercollegiate Guidelines Network (SIGN). Diagnosis and management of epilepsy in adults. Edinburgh (United Kingdom): SIGN; 2015.

26. National Quality Measures Clearinghouse (NCQA). Uses of quality measures. Available at: http://www.qualitymeasures.ahrq.gov/selecting-and-using/using.aspx. Accessed July 6, 2015.

27. Kotter T, Blozik E, Scherer M. Methods for the guideline-based development of quality indicators: a systematic review. Implement Sci 2012;7:21.

28. Brook RH. The RAND/UCLA appropriateness method. Santa Monica (CA): RAND Corporation; 1995.

29. Fountain NB. Delivering quality care in epilepsy. Curr Opin Neurol 2013;26(2): 174–8.

30. Centers for Medicare & Medicaid Services. What information can I get about hospitals?. Medicare.gov/Hospital Compare. 2015. Available at: https://www.medicare.gov/hospitalcompare/About/Hospital-Info.html?AspxAutoDetectCookieSupport=1. Accessed July 6, 2015.

31. Health Affairs. Health policy brief: pay-for-performance. Available at: http://www.healthaffairs.org/healthpolicybriefs/brief.php?brief_id=78. Accessed October 11, 2012.

32. Fountain NB, Van Ness PC, Swain-Eng R, et al. Quality improvement in neurology: AAN epilepsy quality measures: report of the quality measurement and reporting subcommittee of the American Academy of Neurology. Neurology 2011;76(1): 94–9.

33. Centers for Disease Control. Epidemiologic, population, and health outcome studies 2012. Available at: http://www.cdc.gov/epilepsy/research/epi/index.htm. Accessed July 6, 2015.

34. Center for Disease Control and Prevention. Epilepsy in adults and access to care—United States, 2010. MMWR Morb Mortal Wkly Rep 2012;61(45): 909–13. Available at: http://www.cdc.gov/mmwr/preview/mmwrhtml/mm6145a2.htm. Accessed July 6, 2015.

35. Pugh MJ, Berlowitz DR, Montouris G, et al. What constitutes high quality of care for adults with epilepsy? Neurology 2007;69(21):2020–7.

36. Pugh MJ, Berlowitz DR, Rao JK, et al. The quality of care for adults with epilepsy: an initial glimpse using the QUIET measure. BMC Health Serv Res 2011;11(1):1.

37. American Medical Association. About the PCPI. Available at: http://www.ama-assn.org/ama/pub/physician-resources/physician-consortium-performance-improvement/about-pcpi.page?. Accessed July 6, 2015.

38. Pourdeyhimi R, Wolf BJ, Simpson AN, et al. Adherence to outpatient epilepsy quality indicators at a tertiary epilepsy center. Epilepsy Behav 2014;39:26–32.
39. Wicks P, Fountain NB. Patient assessment of physician performance of epilepsy quality-of-care measures. Neurol Clin Pract 2012;2(4):335–42.
40. Ladner TR, Morgan CD, Pomerantz DJ, et al. Does adherence to epilepsy quality measures correlate with reduced epilepsy-related adverse hospitalizations? A retrospective experience. Epilepsia 2015;56(5):e63–7.
41. Kerr EA, Krein SL, Vijan S, et al. Avoiding pitfalls in chronic disease quality measurement: a case for the next generation of technical quality measures. Am J Manag Care 2001;7(11):1033–43.
42. Kerr EA, Smith DM, Hogan MM, et al. Building a better quality measure: are some patients with 'poor quality' actually getting good care? Med Care 2003;41(10): 1173–82.
43. Institute of Medicine. Epilepsy across the spectrum: promoting health and understanding. National Academies Press; 2012.
44. Institute of Medicine. The learning healthcare system. Washington, DC: National Academies Press; 2007.
45. Pugh MJ, Leykum LK, Lanham HJ, et al. Implementation of the epilepsy center of excellence to improve access to and quality of care–protocol for a mixed methods study. Implement Sci 2014;9(1):44.

Guidelines and Quality Standards in the Care of Children with Epilepsy

Martin Kirkpatrick, MBBS, FRCPCH, DCH[a],*,
Colin Dunkley, MBChB, BSc, MRCPCH[b]

KEYWORDS

- Epilepsy • Children • Guidelines • Health services • Quality standards

KEY POINTS

- Clinical practice guidelines allow a synthesis of the best available research evidence into recommendations for best clinical practice.
- Many clinical practice guidelines in children's epilepsy are able to call on only a limited quantitative research base and rely on clinical opinion in formulating recommendations. There may be opportunities to incorporate more qualitative literature into clinical guidance.
- Implementation is vital to ensure that guidelines are translated into improved patient outcomes.

INTRODUCTION

Practice guidelines for clinical care have been in existence in various forms over many years. This article reviews the structures needed to ensure that clinical guidance is based on best available research evidence but also explores the limitations of some of the approaches in particular with regard to epilepsy care in children. Moving the recommendations that emerge from structured clinical guidance into improving quality of care remains a challenge in many health care systems, and the authors review the development of national quality standards, in this case with specific reference to the United Kingdom.

DRIVERS FOR GUIDELINE DEVELOPMENT IN THE UNITED KINGDOM

In the United Kingdom there had been a long-standing concern about the quality of care provided for people with epilepsy, both children and adults. The Chief Medical

Disclosure Statement: The authors have nothing to disclose.
[a] Department of Child Health, University of Dundee, Dundee DD1 9SY, UK; [b] Department of Paediatrics, Sherwood Forest Hospitals, King's Mill Hospital, Sutton in Ashfield, Nottinghamshire NG17 4JL, UK
* Corresponding author.
E-mail address: martin.kirkpatrick@nhs.net

Neurol Clin 34 (2016) 327–337
http://dx.doi.org/10.1016/j.ncl.2015.11.004
0733-8619/16/$ – see front matter © 2016 Elsevier Inc. All rights reserved.

Officer for England commented that epilepsies had remained "in the shadows" for decades, that 5 earlier reports had remained largely unimplemented, and that the disease remained an "unglamorous" area of clinical practice.[1] That this situation is unlikely to have been unique to the United Kingdom has been reflected in the 1997 leading article in *The Lancet* on poorly treated epilepsy.[2]

As examples of this concern, the UK National Clinical Audit of Epilepsy-Related Death reviewed pre-death care and post-death investigations in children and adults over 12 months.[3] Although the proportion of children that could be reviewed in detail was small, the key findings showed that 77% of children had what would be regarded as substandard care and that 59% of deaths in children were potentially or probably avoidable. Deficiencies identified included inadequate drug management, access to specialist care and investigations, and a lack of holistic management.

A report commissioned by the Royal College of Paediatrics and Child Health on the care of children with epilepsies by an individual UK paediatrician was published in 2003. It found that of almost 2000 children with a diagnosis of epilepsy, 32% had been misdiagnosed, either because they did not have epilepsy or the type of epilepsy diagnosed was incorrect. There seemed to be excessive and/or unnecessary drug treatment in almost one-third of children. This doctor's practice is unlikely to have been unique; high rates of misdiagnosis have been reported from elsewhere. For example, of 223 children referred to a tertiary center in Denmark, 85% of which were already on antiepileptic drug treatment, the diagnosis of epilepsy was removed in approximately 40%.[4]

The Royal College of Physicians of Edinburgh convened a conference of interested professionals in Edinburgh in September 2002 leading to the publication of the Edinburgh consensus statement.[5] It noted, for example, that there was an urgent need for national standards of clinical practice to be implemented and monitored. It called on the initial diagnosis of epilepsy to take place in the context of a properly resourced integrated clinical network and for patients to be seen within 2 weeks of referral. The diagnosis of epilepsy should be confirmed by a clinician with expertise in epilepsy as demonstrated by training and continuing education in the epilepsies, peer review of practice, and regular audit of diagnoses. Epilepsies should account for a significant part of this clinician's clinical workload, equivalent to at least one clinic per week.

In large part the development of national guidelines from Scotland (Scottish Intercollegiate Guidelines Network [SIGN]) and from England and Wales (National Institute for Health and Care Excellence [NICE]) arose from these issues.[6,7] It is likely that similar imperatives in other countries have been instrumental in decisions to introduce similar clinical practice guidelines in other countries.

DEFINITIONS OF GUIDELINES

It is nonetheless important to understand what clinical guidelines are and the basis on which they are constructed. Clinical guidelines are defined as *"systematically developed statements to assist practitioner and patient decisions about appropriate health care for specific clinical circumstances."*[8]

However, not all guidelines are systematically developed and in reality may be consensus statements or a position statement by an organization, be they professional, governmental, or lobby. An interested reader looking for published clinical guidance on children's epilepsy might enter the search term *guideline children epilepsy* into a typical Internet search engine. This would reveal some 34,000 results; even using the same search term in a medical scientific journal dedicated to identifying *best practice* literature would identify some 50 guidelines on diagnosis, 84 on treatment, and a further 43 more with generic guidance.[9] The scope of individual guidelines varies hugely, with some addressing narrow areas of a single issue in clinical practice and others attempting to encompass the full breadth of the subject.

When carefully scrutinized it is easily apparent that many guidelines, no less for epilepsy care, struggle to amass robust quantitative evidence and rely on lower levels of evidence including clinical opinion and experience. The purpose of guidelines is to influence practice or policy, in this case, for the care of children with epilepsy. It is often challenging for practicing clinicians to understand and implement what ought to be, as far as is possible, evidence-based practice. Can expert opinion sometimes be confused with clinical evidence?

COMPONENTS OF A SYSTEMATICALLY DEVELOPED CLINICAL PRACTICE GUIDELINE

Several organizations have published guidelines for guidelines setting out the steps and criteria for the development of clinical guidance. These organizations include the World Health Organization, the American Academy of Neurology, National Health and Medical Research Council (Australia), NICE, the SIGN, and the Royal College of Paediatrics and Child Health.[10–14] With the aim of being specific to epilepsy care, the International League Against Epilepsy has recently completed "A Handbook and Tool Kit for Developing Clinical Practice Guidelines".[15] All of these have common themes and most use the Appraisal of Guidelines for Research and Evaluation II (AGREE II) standards, an internationally recognized tool.[16]

The AGREE II tool uses 6 broad headings summarized in **Box 1** (from SIGN 50).[12]

Scope

It is obvious that the overall objective of the guideline should be clear. This objective should include the need for the guideline (the gap in the market). There may be little to be gained in repeating previous similar work already done. An adaptation of an earlier guideline may be a more efficient way of using a guideline in a different geographic or resource context, and tools exist to allow this.[17] Is there evidence of variation in practice that would highlight the need for a guideline? Is it likely that care would be improved for significant numbers in the population? What are the views of patients or users of the service? Is this group of individuals to be covered in the guideline carefully defined? An initial indication of the availability of an evidence base may influence a decision to embark on a formal process.

Developing a series of carefully structured questions is key to the likely success of the guideline process, and without this it is unlikely that clearly defined recommendations can be made. Commonly the PICO format is used to achieve this: defining the Population covered, the Intervention, be it a diagnostic or therapeutic tool, any Comparator intervention, and the Outcome (relevance and measurement).

Stakeholder Involvement

The need for guideline development groups to be multidisciplinary is widely accepted. No clinical guideline that will unambiguously answer every clinical question with a robust and flawless evidence base and to varying degrees will fall back toward consensus for some or part of those questions. A systematic review of factors affecting the judgments produced by formal consensus development methods in health care observed that multi-specialty groups were preferable to single-specialty groupings.[18] Representation of the target audience should be included, and many would suggest that for children and young people the views of that group and that of their parents should be included as an essential part of the process.

Box 1
The 6 broad headings of the AGREE II tool

Scope and purpose

1. The overall objectives of the guideline should be specifically described.

2. The health questions covered by the guideline should be specifically described.

3. The population (patients, public, and so forth) to whom the guideline is meant to apply should be specifically described.

Stakeholder involvement

1. The guideline development group should include individuals from all relevant professional groups.

2. The views and preferences of the target population (patients, public, and so forth) should be sought.

3. The target users of the guideline should be clearly defined.

Rigor of development

1. Systematic methods should be used to search for evidence.

2. The criteria for selecting the evidence should be clearly described.

3. The strengths and limitations of the body of evidence should be clearly described.

4. The methods for formulating the recommendations should be clearly described.

5. The health benefits, side effects, and risks should be considered in formulating the recommendations.

6. There should be an explicit link between the recommendations and the supporting evidence.

7. The guideline should be externally reviewed by experts before publication.

8. A procedure for updating the guideline should be provided.

Clarity of presentation

1. The recommendations should be specific and unambiguous.

2. The different options for management of the condition or health issue should be clearly presented.

3. Key recommendations should be easily identifiable.

Applicability

1. The guideline should describe facilitators and barriers to its application.

2. The guideline should provide advice and/or tools on how the recommendation can be put into practice.

3. The potential cost implications of applying the recommendations should be considered.

4. The guideline should present monitoring and/or auditing criteria.

Editorial independence

1. The views of the funding body should not influence the content of the guideline.

2. Competing interests of guideline development group members should be recorded and addressed.

Adapted from Scottish Intercollegiate Guidelines Network (SIGN). SIGN 50: a guideline developer's handbook. Edinburgh: SIGN; 2014. (SIGN publication no. 50). [October 2014]. Available from URL: http://www.sign.ac.uk.

Guideline Development

Close in importance to precisely structured questions is the formal appraisal of the evidence. The search strategy should explicitly link to those questions. The methodology for identifying, reviewing and synthesizing the evidence should be carefully defined and best practice would suggest that search result is independently scrutinized by 2 reviewers and an appropriate audit trail of the process should be in place. Validated tools exist to appraise systematic reviews and meta-analyses, and an example of this is the PRiSMA (Preferred Reporting Items for Systematic Reviews and Meta-Analyses) tool.[19]

Evidence and Recommendations

The now most widely accepted way of evaluating the strength of the evidence and deriving appropriate recommendations from them is using the GRADE (Grading of Recommendations, Assessment, Development and Evaluations) methodology.[20] It differs from other grading systems in several fundamental ways, including an explicit separation of the quality of evidence and the strength of recommendations. Importantly too, an assessment of the strength of the recommendation is also based on the balance of desirable and undesirable effects, patients' values and preferences, and a consideration of resource utilization. In other words, the quality of the evidence is linked closely into estimates of effectiveness.

Using GRADE, the quality of the evidence is divided into 4 categories: high quality, moderate quality, low quality, and very low quality; but then the criteria described earlier are integrated into an assessment of effectiveness to form either a strong or a weak recommendation. This information is shown in **Table 1**.

In the same way as for many scientific journals, many guideline processes will seek an external peer review of the draft guideline, often seeking views of a range of different experts from different disciplines.

Clarity of Presentation, Applicability, and Editorial Independence

Not only should the recommendations be specific and unambiguous but those that are key should also be clearly identified. When there are different options for management, they should be clearly presented. Issues of implementation and of continuing

Table 1
Determinants of the strength of recommendations

Factor	Considerations
Balance between desirable and undesirable effects	The larger the difference between the desirable and undesirable effects, the higher the likelihood that a strong recommendation is warranted. The narrower the gradient, the higher the likelihood that a weak recommendation is warranted.
Quality of evidence	The higher the quality of evidence, the higher the likelihood that a strong recommendation is warranted.
Values and preferences	The more values and preferences vary, or the greater the uncertainty in values and preferences, the higher the likelihood that a weak recommendation is warranted.
Costs and resource allocation	The higher the cost and resources consumed, the lower the likelihood that a strong recommendation is warranted.

Adapted from Guyatt GH, Oxman AD, Vist GE, et al. GRADE Working Group. GRADE: an emerging consensus on rating quality of evidence and strength of recommendations. BMJ 2008;336(7650):924–6.

audit should be presented in the guideline and potential resource implications of implementing the guidance should be identified. All members of the guideline development group should declare competing interests, and the guideline should be drawn up independent of the views of the funding body.

WEAKNESSES OF THE EVIDENCE-BASED GUIDELINES APPROACH

While recognizing the strength of synthesizing good quality quantitative evidence into robust recommendations for clinical practice, there are several potential weaknesses to this approach (**Box 2**).

Box 2
Weaknesses of the evidence-based guidelines approach

- Clinical questions do not necessarily reflect patient need.
- Clinical questions are in part driven by available published literature.
- There is an effect of bias of clinical opinion in critical assessment of literature.
- Potentially valuable qualitative literature often does not fit into traditional guidelines model.

THE ROLE OF QUALITATIVE LITERATURE: THE LOST TRIBE IN CLINICAL GUIDELINES?

Might we be missing other opportunities to improve care through appraisal of other sources of evidence? As an example, there were 52 guideline recommendations or "good practice points" (the latter derived from the expert opinion of the group) in the SIGN guideline on children's epilepsy. Of these fifty two, 9 were based on appraised evidence from systematic review, randomized control trials, case control, or cohort studies and 29 were based on the consensus opinion of the group. The standardized methodology used in SIGN tends to ignore qualitative or mixed-methods studies except when patient issues were taken into account.[12] Should the status of the randomized controlled trial or meta-analysis remain the sacred cow of clinical practice guidance and perhaps to the exclusion of all else? Many well-structured clinical guidelines will be transparent about the recommendations and on what basis they are founded, and in reality many are based on consensus of the guideline development group. They may well be based on expert and experienced opinion, but the process of literature appraisal has often already sifted out literature that does not meet stringent criteria. Almost all qualitative literature will have been excluded, and the group has no option but to revert down to consensus. In effect, the mass of qualitative literature has been ignored.

In a review of this area, Turner-Stokes and colleagues[21] criticized the applicability and limitations of traditional quantitative research methods in the context of long-term health conditions. The effects of a long-term health condition, such as epilepsy, evolve often over many years and beyond the timescale of many clinical studies. Interventions in the care of children with epilepsy themselves are often long-term and involve multidisciplinary input. Many have complex, interlinked comorbid conditions interacting on a background of an array of social and environmental factors. The investigators are at pains to acknowledge the important role of the typical traditional quantitative methodologies but emphasize the potential contribution of qualitative methodologies. Two reviews comparing the results of observational studies with randomized controlled trials found no evidence of overestimates of the magnitude of treatment effects.[22,23]

The Cochrane Collaboration has attempted to move this issue forward in recent guidance in 2011. Quality assessment of qualitative research studies remains a contested area; but it does set out a framework for the critical appraisal of qualitative studies in informing, enhancing, and extending reviews.[24] Supplementing review whereby qualitative evidence is appraised to address questions other than effectiveness is, however, excluded from Cochrane Intervention reviews. It is proposed that tools for appraisal need to assess quality over several domains, including an assessment of the rigor of reporting and of methodology and ascertaining conceptual breadth and depth. Acknowledging differences in terminology may go some way to allow comparability between qualitative and quantitative research. **Table 2** sets out a proposal to achieve this.

In a systematic review of the contribution of qualitative research to the study of quality of life in children and adolescents with epilepsy, McEwan and colleagues[25] retrieved 17 studies. They varied significantly in their quality, but a third had used some form of systematically developed qualitative or mixed methods methodology and were able to draw valid conclusions from this literature.

In a further mixed-methods systematic review, Lewis and colleagues[26] reviewed the knowledge and information needs of young people with epilepsy aged 13 to 19 years. The filtering process took 434 citations down to 40 studies of which 19 met inclusion criteria for the review. There was a consistent emerging message about the inadequacy of information provision and exchange in young people, an issue that would be very unlikely to have been considered in any quantitative study.

Much qualitative literature probably remains an untapped source of information to be synthesized into improving standards of care in children's epilepsy.

GUIDELINE IMPLEMENTATION

The implementation of a guideline should be seen as an ongoing, continuous, and integrated component of the guideline development and redevelopment process. A formal blueprint of recommended practice is only really an initial, albeit vital, first step in a process that is ultimately aiming to optimize quality of care and clinical outcomes for each individual in the target population. Difficulties with implementation can begin soon after publication. Some who have been involved in guideline production may have experienced a sense that the publication of a guideline marked the end of the process and an impression that the guideline will implement itself. On the receiving end, the necessary next steps of implementation can vary wildly from thinking *thankfully, this is what we can prove we are already doing* to *these recommendations are so aspirational that they are not possible to implement*—marking 2 extremes.

With regard to epilepsy, there are particular inherent aspects that make implementation difficult (**Box 3**).

Table 2 Criteria to critically appraise findings from qualitative research		
Aspect	**Qualitative Term**	**Quantitative Term**
Truth value	Credibility	Internal validity
Applicability	Transferability	External validity or generalizability
Consistency	Dependability	Reliability
Neutrality	Confirmability	Objectivity

Adapted from Concato J, Shah N, Horwitz RI. Randomized, controlled trials, observational studies, and the hierarchy of research designs. N Engl J Med 2000;342(25):1887–92.

Box 3
Guideline implementation difficulties for epilepsy

- Epilepsies are a group of heterogeneous conditions, and what constitutes best practice for one child may vary considerably from what constitutes best practice for another.

- The patient journey for an individual child is likely to involve acute and non-acute care and different health and non-health professionals.

- The optimum clinical outcomes for children with epilepsy are not always easily definable or measurable and will include quality of life, developmental and educational outcomes, as well as seizure control and adverse effects.

- Clinical decision making and appraisal of risk-benefit for individual patients with epilepsy are not easily captured in an epilepsy guideline. To do so requires a degree of expertise, and working to a guideline is not the same as applying expertise.

The "Handbook and Tool Kit for Developing Clinical Practice Guidelines"[15] emphasizes how implementation can be considered throughout the guideline development process. It highlights studies demonstrating low levels of professional awareness of guidelines and revealing poor adoption of guidelines.

The following elements of this article consider the implementation process in more detail and in particular example the UK experience of implementation continuing since the NICE and SIGN guideline publication some 12 years ago.

Dissemination

Following guideline publication the guideline should be actively and freely made available to all relevant parties. Many guidelines are now produced in different formats according to their intended recipients, for example, electronic versus printed, full versus abridged, and commissioner versus practitioner versus patient formats. Dissemination may include a package of other resources, including archiving of earlier versions, gap analysis tools, presentation slides, display posters, and audit tools.

Guideline Appraisal

For many, guideline implementation will begin by reading and appraising the guideline. The next steps will then depend on an individual's professional roles and responsibilities. Ideally all within a health community will realize they have one or several roles to play in different aspects of guideline implementation. A gap analysis or baseline assessment is a useful first step in highlighting relevant recommendations within a guideline that need action. Some will have several roles when considering a guideline. How should my personal practice change? How should this inform the development of my team's service? How should this inform my regional or network working? How should this now align with national strategies and interventions? The ADAPTE process is a comprehensive tool kit aiming to translate one guideline into a consistent locally applicable and acceptable guideline.[17]

United Kingdom case study

NICE and SIGN published guidance for the management of epilepsy in childhood in 2004 and 2005, respectively.[6,7] As well as containing recommendations regarding assessment, diagnosis, investigation, and treatment, they outlined referral pathways, roles and competences of different types of professionals, prolonged convulsion protocols, and liaison with education and mental health services. It was acknowledged from the outset that implementation would require more than effecting change in personal practice.

Education and Training

In 2005, the British Paediatric Neurology Association commissioned a portfolio of standardized Paediatric Epilepsy Training (PET) courses. Each PET course is aimed at different types of nurses and doctors and includes clear learning aims and objectives. The courses encourage grey-case application of guidance and peer-to-peer learning via an interactive case-based workshop style. These courses have explicitly embedded NICE and SIGN recommendations within their educational spine and course materials.

Workforce Planning

NICE and SIGN guidance has also emphasized the importance of appropriate expertise in applying clinical care. Particular emphasis was made regarding the role of the paediatrician with expertise in epilepsies and the epilepsy specialist nurse. The competences required for these roles have been further defined via the Royal College of Nursing[27] and the Royal College of Paediatrics and Child Health.[28] Definitions of such roles along defined pathways within clear populations allow the potential for clear service specifications and workforce planning.

Quality Standards

In 2013, NICE published 9 quality standards for paediatric epilepsy.[29] These standards are defined quality measures derived directly from key guidelines. These standardized metrics allow services to measure the success of guideline implementation and, thereby, a perspective on the quality of care delivered.

Audit and Benchmarking

Audit describes the ongoing process of improving actual care delivered toward recommended practice. Since the launch of UK guidance the audit of epilepsies in the UK has evolved from locally developed audit toward repeating cycles of systematic standardized UK audit. Epilepsy12 (a UK national audit measuring 12 clinical performance indicators over 12 months) received funding to facilitate a UK wide audit of practice against NICE and SIGN recommendations for all relevant paediatric providers. The audit comprised 3 domains: a census and mapping of UK service configurations, 12 clinical performance indicators from a carefully ascertained cohort of new patients, and a series of patient-reported experience measures. In 2012, the first Epilepsy12 report showed gaps and variations in care. In 2014, the second Epilepsy12 audit published longitudinal data demonstrating continuing variation but statistically significant widespread improvements in quality of care. The audit required individuals, services, and commissioners to undertake action plans and follow recommendations tailored around practice-dependent and resource-dependent factors.[30]

Clinical Networks

Some of the published concerns regarding quality of care in the United Kingdom have stemmed from professionals working in isolation. Many children with epilepsy require professionals working together who have clearly defined shared care arrangements, common resources, and agreed pathways of care from local care to regional or national centers. Clinical networks provide a visible forum for groups of professionals to work collaboratively to improve care. Examples of network functions include discussion of complex cases, benchmarking and sharing of quality improvements, development of regional patient information resources, educational programs, and so forth.

SUMMARY

There is emerging formal consensus regarding what constitutes best practice for children and young people with epilepsy. However, this is an ongoing process that needs to provoke and keep up with an expanding evidence base. There remains much to learn and much to do. In the same way that primary research needs rigor and expertise, so does the process of guideline development and guideline implementation. Good science can then lead to good clinical practice recommendations and then, crucially, lead further to good clinical outcomes.

REFERENCES

1. The annual report of the Chief Medical Officer of the Department of Health 2001. Available at: http://www.dh.gov.uk/prod_consum_dh/groups/dh_digitalassets/@dh/@en/documents/digitalasset/dh_4082273.pdf. Accessed July 1, 2015.
2. In the shadow of epilepsy. Lancet 1997;349(9069):1851.
3. Hanna NJ, Black M, Sander JW, et al. National sentinel clinical audit of epilepsy-related death: epilepsy – death in the shadows. London: The Stationery Office; 2002.
4. Uldall P, Alving J, Hansen LK, et al. The misdiagnosis of epilepsy in children admitted to a tertiary epilepsy centre with paroxysmal events. Arch Dis Child 2006;91:219–21.
5. Consensus statement on better care for children and adults with epilepsy. J R Coll Physicians Edinb 2003;33(Suppl 11):2–3.
6. Scottish Intercollegiate Guidelines Network. Diagnosis and management of epilepsies in children and young people (SIGN 81). Edinburgh (United Kingdom): SIGN; 2005.
7. National Institute for Health and Clinical Excellence. Epilepsies: diagnosis and management. Clinical Guideline 137. London: NICE; 2012.
8. Woolf SH, Grol R, Hutchinson A, et al. Clinical guidelines: potential benefits, limitations, and harms of clinical guidelines. BMJ 1999;318(7182):527–30.
9. Available at: http://bestpractice.bmj.com/best-practice/search.html?searchableText=epilepsy+and+children&aliasHandle=guidelines&languageCode=en. Accessed July 1, 2015.
10. World Health Organization, editor. WHO handbook for guideline development. Geneva (Switzerland): World Health Organization; 2012.
11. Gronseth GS, Woodroffe LM, Getchius TS. Clinical practice guideline process manual. St. Paul (MN): American Academy of Neurology; 2011.
12. SIGN. SIGN 50: a guideline developer's handbook. Edinburgh (United Kingdom): SIGN; 2011.
13. NICE. The guidelines manual. London: NICE; 2012.
14. Higgins JPT, Green S. Cochrane Handbook for Systematic Reviews of Interventions Version 5.1.0 [updated March 2011]. Oxford: The Cochrane Collaboration; 2011.
15. Sauro KM, Wiebe S, Perucca E, et al. Developing clinical practice guidelines for epilepsy: A report from the ILAE Epilepsy Guidelines Working Group. Epilepsia 2015;56(12):1859–69.
16. Brouwers MC, Kho ME, Browman GP, et al. AGREE II: advancing guideline development, reporting and evaluation in health care. CMAJ 2010;182(18):E839–42.
17. Available at: http://www.g-i-n.net/working-groups/adaptation. Accessed July 1, 2015.

18. Hutchings A, Raine R. A systematic review of factors affecting the judgments produced by formal consensus development methods in health care. J Health Serv Res Policy 2006;11(3):172–9.
19. Moher D, Liberati A, Tetzlaff J, et al. Preferred reporting items for systematic reviews and meta-analyses: the PRISMA statement. Int J Surg 2010;8(5):336–41.
20. Handbook for grading the quality of evidence and the strength of the recommendations using the GRADE approach. Available at: http://www.guidelinedevelopment.org/handbook/2013. Accessed July 1, 2015.
21. Turner-Stokes L, Harding R, Sergeant J, et al. Generating the evidence base for the national service framework for long term conditions: a new research typology. Clin Med 2006;6(1):91–7.
22. Benson K, Hartz AJ. A comparison of observational studies and randomized, controlled trials. N Engl J Med 2000;342(25):1878–86.
23. Concato J, Shah N, Horwitz RI. Randomized, controlled trials, observational studies, and the hierarchy of research designs. N Engl J Med 2000;342(25): 1887–92.
24. Hannes K. Critical appraisal of qualitative research. In: Noyes J, Booth A, Hannes K, et al, editors. Supplementary guidance for inclusion of qualitative research in Cochrane systematic reviews of interventions. Version 1. Oxford: Cochrane Collaboration Qualitative Methods Group; 2011. Available at: http://cqrmg.cochrane.org/supplemental-handbook-guidance.
25. McEwan MJ, Espie CA, Metcalfe J. A systematic review of the contribution of qualitative research to the study of quality of life in children and adolescents with epilepsy. Seizure 2004;13(1):3–14.
26. Lewis SA, Noyes J, Mackereth S, et al. Knowledge and information needs of young people with epilepsy and their parents: mixed-method systematic review. BMC Pediatr 2010;10:103.
27. Royal College of Nursing. Specialist nursing of children and young people with epilepsy. RCN guidance for service planning and career development. London: RCN Publications; 2013.
28. Royal College of Paediatrics and Child Health. A framework of competences for level 3 special study module in paediatric epilepsies. London: RCPCH publications; 2013.
29. National Institute for Health and Clinical Excellence. The epilepsies in children and young people. Quality Standards 27. London: National Institute for Health and Care Excellence; 2013.
30. Royal College of Paediatrics and Child Health. Epilepsy12 national report. Round 2. London: RCPCH Publications; 2012.

Initial Evaluation of the Patient with Suspected Epilepsy

Nathalie Jetté, MD, MSc, FRCPC[a,b], Samuel Wiebe, MD, MSc, FRCPC[a,b],*

KEYWORDS

- Definition of epilepsy • Newly diagnosed • Misdiagnosis • Differential diagnosis
- Investigation • Referral • Psychiatric comorbidity • Neuro-cognitive outcomes

KEY POINTS

- Epilepsy can be diagnosed after a single unprovoked seizure if a patient's risk of having a recurrent seizure is similar to that after 2 unprovoked seizures (>60%).
- Predictors of recurrent seizure include a previous brain injury, a significant abnormality on brain imaging, and a seizure occurring out of sleep.
- An epilepsy specialist who can promptly establish the diagnosis should see patients with new-onset seizures.
- An electroencephalogram is recommended in those with suspected or newly diagnosed epilepsy. Brain imaging (preferably MRI) is recommended in those with new-onset unprovoked seizures unless they have a clear generalized epilepsy of genetic origin.
- Patients with new-onset epilepsy should be screened for depression and anxiety, and undergo neurocognitive testing when appropriate.

INTRODUCTION

Receiving a diagnosis of new-onset epilepsy can be life changing. Epilepsy is associated with a number of poor outcomes, including premature mortality, multimorbidity, and social and psychosocial challenges, such as driving restrictions,

Disclosures: N. Jetté holds a Canada Research Chair in Neurological Health Services Research. S. Wiebe holds the Hopewell Professorship of Clinical Neurosciences Research at the University of Calgary. The authors have no commercial or financial conflicts of interest.
[a] Department of Clinical Neurosciences, Hotchkiss Brain Institute, Foothills Medical Centre, Cumming School of Medicine, University of Calgary, 1403 29 Street Northwest, Room C1209, Calgary, Alberta T2N 2T9, Canada; [b] Department of Community Health Sciences, O'Brien Institute for Public Health, Foothills Medical Centre, Cumming School of Medicine, University of Calgary, 1403 29 Street Northwest, Room C1209, Calgary, Alberta T2N 2T9, Canada
* Corresponding author. Department of Clinical Neurosciences, Hotchkiss Brain Institute, Foothills Medical Centre, Cumming School of Medicine, University of Calgary, 1403 29 Street Northwest, Room C1209, Calgary, Alberta T2N 2T9, Canada.
E-mail address: swiebe@ucalgary.ca

Neurol Clin 34 (2016) 339–350
http://dx.doi.org/10.1016/j.ncl.2015.11.008
0733-8619/16/$ – see front matter © 2016 Elsevier Inc. All rights reserved.

unemployment, and stigma.[1-3] As such, the prompt evaluation of those who present with possible epilepsy is necessary to ensure they are accurately diagnosed and properly managed. Important new concepts have emerged in recent years, including that epilepsy can now be diagnosed after a single unprovoked seizure under certain circumstances. There is also a new classification of seizures and the epilepsies, along with a definition of drug-resistant epilepsy that should promote an earlier referral to specialized epilepsy programs. We review the approach to the initial evaluation of the person with suspected epilepsy, including new definitions, which diagnostic tests should be considered, and when early referral to an epilepsy program is suggested.

IS IT EPILEPSY?
Definition of Epilepsy

Epilepsy has traditionally been defined as a "condition characterized by recurrent (2 or more) epileptic seizures, unprovoked by any immediate cause."[4] However, it has become evident to experts over time that there are instances in which a single seizure may signal the presence of epilepsy. Indeed, in 2005, the following conceptual definition of epilepsy was proposed by the International League Against Epilepsy (ILAE) and the International Bureau for Epilepsy, although it was not initially adopted: "Epilepsy is a disorder of the brain characterized by an enduring predisposition to generate epileptic seizures and by the neurobiologic, cognitive, psychosocial, and social consequences of this condition. The definition of epilepsy requires the occurrence of at least one epileptic seizure."[5] Although some were concerned by the risks of diagnosing epilepsy after a single seizure (eg, stigma in those who may not go on to have epilepsy), others also saw merit in this proposal. Earlier identification of those with suspected epilepsy could (1) reduce the time to intervention and as a result decrease injuries and morbidity, (2) provide the opportunity to introduce disease-modifying therapies when available, and (3) allow for the prevention or the earlier assessment and management of comorbidities with the goal of improving overall epilepsy-related outcomes. A few years ago, the ILAE commissioned a task force to convert this conceptual definition into a practical definition that could be used for clinical care. The new definition of epilepsy (**Box 1**) was adopted by the ILAE Executive Committee in December 2013, after undergoing extensive review (public comments by more than 200 individuals, journal reviewers, and so forth).[6] The most significant change to the classic epilepsy definition is the adoption of the concept that epilepsy can now be diagnosed in a patient with reflex seizures and after a single seizure, if the patient's risk of having a recurrent seizure is similar to that after 2 unprovoked seizures, which is at least 60%.

Box 1
Practical clinical definition of epilepsy

Epilepsy is a disorder of the brain defined by any of the following conditions

1. At least 2 unprovoked (or reflex) seizures occurring more than 24 hours apart

2. One unprovoked (or reflex) seizure and a probability of further seizures similar to the general recurrence risk (at least 60%) after 2 unprovoked seizures, occurring over the next 10 years

Adapted from Fisher RS, Acevedo C, Arzimanoglou A, et al. ILAE official report: a practical clinical definition of epilepsy. Epilepsia 2014;55:477; with permission.

When Can We Say Someone Has Epilepsy After a Single Seizure?

The risk of a second seizure after a single unprovoked seizure is between 24% and 65%,[7] and the risk after 2 unprovoked seizures is 73% at 4 years. However, determining in which cases a single seizure may herald epilepsy is more challenging, although in general the risk is greater than 60% in those with a history of remote or subacute stroke, central nervous system infection, or trauma.[8] Guidance in determining the risk of recurrent seizure may be obtained by using a prognostic index derived from the Medical Research Council Multicenter Trial for Early Epilepsy and Single Seizure (MESS) Study, whereby a history of both neurologic disorder or deficit, learning disability or developmental delay, AND an abnormal electroencephalogram (EEG) is associated with a greater than 60% risk of recurrent seizure at 3 and 5 years.[9] The new evidence-based guidelines on the management of an unprovoked first seizure in adults also provide guidance with regard to variables that are associated with a greater recurrence risk after a first unprovoked seizure.[10] Predictors of a recurrent seizure after a first unprovoked seizure include a previous brain injury (Level A), an EEG with epileptiform discharges (Level A), a significant abnormality on brain imaging (Level B), and a seizure occurring out of sleep (Level B).[10] The overall impact of the new epilepsy diagnostic criteria is unknown at this time; however, it is exciting to imagine that one could intervene sooner to reduce the morbidity associated with epilepsy. At the same time, the impact of diagnosing epilepsy after a single seizure is unknown in terms of epidemiologic estimates of epilepsy, reimbursement programs, legislation and health economics (eg, driving, insurance coverage), and the economic, social, and emotional consequences on the patient.

How Do You Diagnose Epilepsy?

The National Institute for Health and Care Excellence (NICE) in the United Kingdom provides useful guidance on the initial diagnosis of those with suspected seizure and epilepsy, along with care pathways.[11] The American Academy of Neurology (AAN) has also produced guidelines for the evaluation and management of patients presenting with a first seizure.[10,12] Salient aspects of the NICE and AAN recommendations are summarized in **Fig. 1**. These emphasize clarification of the diagnosis, prompt referral to a specialist with expertise in the management of seizures, performing key initial diagnostic tests, and an individualized approach to management.[11] This recommended approach to the initial evaluation of the patient with suspected seizures is important, as the differential diagnosis of epileptic seizures is broad, and can include provoked seizures (eg, due to hypoglycemia), nonepileptic psychogenic spells, and other physiologic events (eg, migraine, syncope, transient ischemic attacks, tics, rapid eye movement sleep intrusions). The prevalence of epilepsy misdiagnosis is high, reported to range between 16% and 42% depending on the study. Most commonly, patients who are incorrectly diagnosed as having epileptic seizures actually have nonepileptic psychogenic events or syncope.[13] **Table 1** provides the key differentiating features between bilateral convulsive seizure, nonepileptic psychogenic spells, and syncope. The diagnostic tools used to confirm or refute a diagnosis of epilepsy are discussed in the "Role of investigations" section.

How Do We Classify Seizures and Epilepsy Syndromes?

Once a diagnosis of epileptic seizure or epilepsy is made, the next step is to classify the seizure(s) and epilepsy syndrome according to the new ILAE classification and terminology.[14] Seizures are now classified according to whether they are focal, generalized, or unknown and then further defined based on their semiology (**Table 2**).[14] For

Suspected Epilepsy

Obtain detailed history of semiology and identify criteria for definition of Epilepsy

Urgent diagnosis by specialist with expertise in epilepsy

Establish
Seizure type, epilepsy syndrome, cause and comorbidities

EEG
Higher yield if done early after a seizure
Helps support diagnosis
Determine risk of recurrence
Determine type of seizure and epilepsy

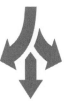

MRI
Obtain in adult onset epilepsy and suspected focal epilepsy
Helps determine risk of recurrence, and need for urgent intervention

Other
Psychosocial assessment
Neuro-Cognitive evaluation
Specific investigations as indicated

Consider Providing
A comprehensive management plan, resources for information needs of patient and caregivers, an individualized approach to the decision to start AEDs, early referral to tertiary care if needed, regular and structured follow-up

Fig. 1. Initial evaluation of patients with suspected epilepsy.

example, a patient formerly thought to have a complex partial seizure beginning with an aura evolving to a secondary generalized tonic-clonic seizure would now be referred to as having focal seizures with aura and dyscognitive features evolving to bilateral convulsive activity (see **Table 2**). In addition, the old terms idiopathic, symptomatic, and cryptogenic are no longer recommended. **Table 3** provides the new terminology that is recommended when classifying an epilepsy according to its etiology. As such, a patient with juvenile myoclonic epilepsy could be classified as having an epilepsy of presumed genetic origin, whereas an older man with new-onset epilepsy after a remote stroke would be classified as having an epilepsy of structural origin.

ROLE OF INVESTIGATIONS IN PATIENTS WITH SUSPECTED EPILEPSY
General Role of Investigations

The patient with suspected epilepsy typically presents with a history of one or more transient episodes of neurologic dysfunction whose clinical features indicate the

Table 1
Features differentiating convulsive seizures from its common mimics

Clinical Feature	Bilateral Convulsive Seizure	Psychogenic Seizure	Syncope
Age	Any	Most common in middle age, but described from childhood to late adulthood	Any
Family history	Occasionally	Rare	Occasionally
Triggers	Usually none except for reflex epilepsy, but sometimes can be triggered by sleep deprivation, stress, nonadherence to AEDs, acute illness, menstrual cycle (ovulation, menses)	Often in the setting of an emotional event; can at times be provoked by suggestion	Change in posture to upright position, venipuncture, painful or noxious stimuli, emotional stress, micturition, Valsalva maneuver
Timing of event	From wakefulness or sleep	Always during wakefulness, usually in the presence of a witness	Almost universally from wakefulness
Clinical features			
Duration	Brief	Prolonged	Brief
Stereotypic	Usually	No	Usually
Onset (aura?)	Usually with abrupt loss of consciousness; occasionally preceded by aura (eg, rising epigastric sensation, smell of burned toast)	Usually (eg, anxiety, upset feeling)	Frequent (eg, dizziness, nausea, visual blurring, lightheadedness)
Motor activity	Generalized tonic stiffening, fall, followed by convulsive activity (very rare to see eye closure)	+/− avoidance behavior, eye closure, irregular limb movements, opisthotonus, pelvic thrusting, rigidity, side-to-side head movements	+/− loss of tone, brief tonic stiffening, brief multifocal myoclonic jerk
Associated features	+/− cyanosis, tongue biting, urinary incontinence, postictal confusion or drowsiness up to hours (usually minutes), headache, myalgia	+/− urinary incontinence (rare), postictal crying	+/− urinary incontinence (rare), rapid recovery, brief postictal confusion if present (usually <30 s)

(continued on next page)

Table 1
(*continued*)

Clinical Feature	Bilateral Convulsive Seizure	Psychogenic Seizure	Syncope
Physical injury	Occasional	Rare	Rare
Investigations			
EEG	Usually abnormal	Normal	Normal
MRI	Frequently abnormal	Normal	Normal
Response to AED therapy	70% respond to treatment	No response to AEDs	No response to AEDs

Abbreviations: AED, antiepileptic drug; EEG, electroencephalogram.
From Wiebe S, Jette N. Pharmacoresistance and the role of surgery in difficult to treat epilepsy. Nat Rev Neurol 2012;8:673; with permission.

possibility of seizures. A detailed, directed clinical history obtained by an experienced clinician from the patient and reliable witnesses remains the diagnostic cornerstone in epilepsy.[15,16] The history will help determine the probability that the events in question are seizures, assess the risk of their recurrence, and confirm or refute the diagnosis of suspected epilepsy with a high level of confidence. Therefore, a specialist with expertise in epilepsy who can establish the diagnosis should see patients with a new onset of seizures or suspected epilepsy as soon as possible.

The role of investigations in patients with an early diagnosis of epilepsy can be conceptualized under 4 major categories: as an extension of the initial assessment

Table 2
Seizure classification according to the ILAE revised terminology for organization of seizures

Seizure Type	Seizure Subtype	Further Possible Seizure Subtype
Generalized seizures	Tonic-clonic	—
	Absence	• Typical • Atypical • With special features (eg, myoclonic absence or eyelid myoclonia)
	Clonic	—
	Tonic	—
	Atonic	—
	Myoclonic	• Myoclonic • Myoclonic-atonic • Myoclonic-tonic
Focal seizures	• With aura • With motor features • With autonomic features • With altered awareness (dys-cognitive features) • Without dyscognitive features	• Evolving to bilateral convulsive seizure
Unknown seizure type	• Epileptic spasms • Other	—

Adapted from Berg AT, Berkovic SF, Brodie MJ, et al. Revised terminology and concepts for organization of seizures and epilepsies: report of the ILAE Commission on Classification and Terminology, 2005–2009. Epilepsia 2010;51:676–85.

Table 3	
Current and past terminology and concept for epilepsy etiology	
Current Terminology and Concept (2010)	**Past Terminology and Concept (1989)**
Genetic	*Idiopathic*
A genetic defect contributes directly to the epilepsy and seizures are the core symptom of this disorder For example, juvenile myoclonic epilepsy	Presumed genetic
Structural-metabolic	*Symptomatic*
A distinct structural or metabolic condition is responsible for the epilepsy For example, epilepsy due to a remote stroke	Secondary to a known or presumed disorder of the brain
Unknown	*Cryptogenic*
The cause is unknown and might be genetic, structural, or metabolic	Presumed symptomatic

Adapted from Berg AT, Berkovic SF, Brodie MJ, et al. Revised terminology and concepts for organization of seizures and epilepsies: report of the ILAE Commission on Classification and Terminology, 2005–2009. Epilepsia 2010;51:676–85.

of the patient, to help determine the type of seizure and epilepsy syndrome, to guide therapy, and to assess prognosis with regard to pharmacoresistance and early considerations of surgical therapy.

Initial Assessment

The rationale and diagnostic yield of initial investigations in patients with suspected epilepsy or first seizures is summarized in **Table 4**. An EEG should be obtained in all patients with suspected or newly diagnosed epilepsy.[11] On average, the EEG demonstrates significant abnormalities (such as epileptiform discharges) in 29% of adults after a first seizure,[12] and it is most sensitive when performed early after seizures. On the other hand, an EEG should not be used as the only means of diagnosing epilepsy or to exclude the diagnosis of epilepsy.[11] Brain imaging (computed tomography or MRI) demonstrates relevant abnormalities in approximately 10% of patients with a first seizure[12] and helps establish the risk of recurrence and therefore the diagnosis of epilepsy after a single seizure. MRI is the preferred imaging method and should be performed early, particularly in the presence of focal abnormalities in the neurologic examination or EEG. On the other hand, imaging is not routinely indicated for patients in whom the diagnosis of genetic (primary) generalized epilepsy is clear (eg, juvenile myoclonic epilepsy, childhood absence epilepsy).[11]

Determining the Type of Seizure and Epilepsy

The type of seizure (see **Table 2**) is generally established based on the clinical semiology. However, a routine EEG can be very helpful in determining the distribution of epileptiform discharges, which provides an indicator of whether seizures are generalized or focal, and if focal, the location of the irritative zone and potentially also the epileptogenic zone. Sleep EEGs or sleep-deprived EEGs increase the yield and should be considered if the routine EEG is not informative.[11] The type of epileptiform discharges in the EEG also helps determine the subtype of epilepsy (eg, focal temporal lobe epilepsy, or generalized epilepsy with absence seizures). Finally, if the EEG captures clinical events, it can also help determine whether the seizures are epileptic or nonepileptic, and if epileptic, the type and location of the seizures. The MRI is of

Table 4
Investigations in adults with a first seizure or suspected epilepsy

Investigation	Estimates and Findings	Comments
Imaging (preferably MRI)	10% have significant abnormalities	Perform early, especially if focal findings. Not routinely in clear genetic generalized epilepsy.
EEG	29% have significant abnormalities	Perform early, to support epilepsy, clarify type of seizure and epilepsy. Not only as grounds for diagnosis of epilepsy; not to rule out epilepsy.
Blood glucose, blood cell count, electrolytes	<5% abnormal in general	May be useful in specific clinical situations with comorbid conditions, but not routinely helpful.
12-lead electrocardiogram	Significant conduction or repolarization defects	NICE recommends routinely for adults with epilepsy. Helpful to assess cardiac risk factors for mortality.
Psychosocial assessment	OR in epilepsy compared with general population for anxiety 2.4, suicidality 2.2, major depression 2.3	Impact adversely on quality of life. Early detection and intervention indicated.
Neurocognitive testing	Wide range of cognitive deficits in focal and generalized epilepsies	Assessment indicated if cognitive dysfunction is identified, or imaging abnormalities involve structures with cognitive representation.
Toxicology screen, lumbar puncture	Low yield	Only in specific circumstances guided by clinical context (eg, suspect CNS infection, intoxication).

Abbreviations: CNS, central nervous system; EEG, electroencephalogram; OR, odds ratios.
Data from Refs.[11,12,17]

particular importance to identify focal lesions, which can lead to the diagnosis of focal epilepsy if supported by corresponding clinical semiology.

Guiding Therapy and Prognosis

The treatment of epilepsy is guided in the first instance by the type of seizure and the type of epilepsy. The EEG and MRI have important roles in this regard by helping determine whether patients require a medication that is targeted primarily at focal or generalized seizures, or at a specific type of epilepsy, such as juvenile myoclonic epilepsy or absence epilepsy. An abnormal EEG also has important prognostic implications. In a classic meta-analysis of people with an initial seizure, the risk of recurrence (and therefore the diagnosis of epilepsy and potential need for therapy) was 1.2 to 4.1 times higher if the EEG showed relevant abnormalities[7]; and the risk was almost twice as high if the abnormalities were epileptiform as opposed to nonepileptiform.[7] In addition, the MRI is instrumental in identifying lesions that require additional assessment, such as vascular lesions and tumors, as well as those that entail a high risk of seizure recurrence or pharmacoresistance and may warrant early evaluation for epilepsy surgery (eg, tumors, hemorrhagic lesions, malformations of cortical development).

PSYCHOLOGICAL AND COGNITIVE ASSESSMENT
Psychological Evaluation

Psychiatric comorbidities are relevant at the time of diagnosis of epilepsy because they are highly prevalent in people with epilepsy,[17] they may predate the diagnosis of epilepsy, and there is mounting evidence that they negatively affect quality of life in children[18] and adults.[19] Furthermore, psychiatric comorbidities remain undetected or untreated in many patients.[20] Therefore, patients with early-onset or suspected epilepsy should be screened for common psychiatric comorbidities such as depression and anxiety, and if present they should be treated. Also, patients and their caregivers should be given information about psychological issues often surrounding epilepsy. Management principles for various neuropsychiatric problems in epilepsy have been put forward by an international consensus group of the ILAE.[21]

Neurocognitive Assessment

Patients with focal and generalized epilepsies are more likely than the general population to have a range of cognitive difficulties, including deficits of language, memory, learning, attention, and executive function.[22] These deficits may predate the diagnosis of epilepsy. For example, attention-deficit/hyperactivity disorder is 2.5 times more common in patients who eventually experience a first seizure than in those who do not.[23] Furthermore, antiepileptic drugs can cause or exacerbate some of these problems, especially with polytherapy or if higher dosages are used. Neurocognitive testing is recommended early on in patients with evidence of language, learning, or memory difficulties, or when MRI shows abnormalities in brain regions involved in cognitive function,[11] so as to intervene appropriately.

ROLE OF EARLY REFERRAL TO SPECIALIZED CENTERS

NICE recommends that patients of any age with suspected seizures or epilepsy be referred to a specialist with expertise in the management of seizures promptly, to confirm the diagnosis and ensure these patients are appropriately investigated and treated.[11] In addition, patients should be referred early to specialized centers if (1) investigations reveal features that indicate a risk of developing drug resistance (defined as failure to control seizures after adequate trials of 2 appropriately used medications in monotherapy or in combination[24]), such as the presence of lesions known to respond poorly to therapy (eg, malformations of cortical development, strokes, and hemosiderin-containing lesions); (2) if patients are experiencing or are at risk of experiencing unacceptable side effects from medications; (3) if patients have a clinically important lesion on imaging; (4) if patients have psychological or mental health comorbidity; or (5) if the diagnosis remains in doubt.[11]

There is also guidance regarding when a patient (whether a child or an adult) should be referred for an epilepsy surgery evaluation.[13,25–27] Referral should be considered for patients whose seizures are drug resistant, as outlined previously.[24] It also has been suggested that any patient with a complex epilepsy syndrome or requiring complex surgery, those with consistently lateralized seizures that cannot be clearly assigned to a definite electroclinical syndrome, children with a lesion that is surgically accessible regardless of seizure frequency, and any child younger than 3 years be referred for evaluation of epilepsy surgery.[27,28] A freely accessible online tool (www.toolsforepilepsy.com) is also available to provide guidance as to when should a patient (age 5 and older) be referred for an epilepsy surgery evaluation (7–8 questions that take approximately 1 minute to complete).[29,30] Although the ideal time to refer for an epilepsy surgery evaluation remains to be determined, a recent randomized controlled trial, the ERSET (Early surgical therapy for drug-resistant temporal lobe epilepsy) trial, found that surgery within 2 years after the onset of drug-resistant epilepsy was superior to ongoing medical management.[31] Cohort studies also confirm the benefit of earlier age at surgery and shorter epilepsy duration before surgery. Timely surgery is associated with better neuropsychiatric, psychiatric, and social outcomes, and is particularly critical in children, in whom it may prevent the development of long-standing psychosocial and cognitive difficulties.[27,32]

SUMMARY

The initial evaluation of the patient with possible new-onset epilepsy is important. Patients under certain circumstances can now be diagnosed with epilepsy after a single seizure, which may in the future allow for the earlier use of neuroprotective agents and the prevention of poor outcomes. The accurate and early identification of seizure and epilepsy types, guided by diagnostic investigations and an epilepsy specialist evaluation, allows for the most appropriate therapeutic approaches to be implemented. However, the initial evaluation of those with suspected epilepsy goes beyond just defining seizure types and the epilepsy syndromes, as it is equally important to ensure epilepsy comorbidity is also carefully screened for and treated.

REFERENCES

1. Nevalainen O, Ansakorpi H, Simola M, et al. Epilepsy-related clinical characteristics and mortality: a systematic review and meta-analysis. Neurology 2014;83: 1968–77.
2. Fiest KM, Birbeck GL, Jacoby A, et al. Stigma in epilepsy. Curr Neurol Neurosci Rep 2014;14:444.
3. Kobau R, Cui W, Kadima N, et al. Tracking psychosocial health in adults with epilepsy—estimates from the 2010 National Health Interview Survey. Epilepsy Behav 2014;41:66–73.
4. Guidelines for epidemiologic studies on epilepsy. Commission on Epidemiology and Prognosis, International League Against Epilepsy. Epilepsia 1993; 34:592–6.
5. Fisher RS, van Emde Boas W, Blume W, et al. Epileptic seizures and epilepsy: definitions proposed by the International League Against Epilepsy (ILAE) and the International Bureau for Epilepsy (IBE). Epilepsia 2005;46:470–2.
6. Fisher RS, Acevedo C, Arzimanoglou A, et al. ILAE official report: a practical clinical definition of epilepsy. Epilepsia 2014;55:475–82.
7. Berg AT, Shinnar S. The risk of seizure recurrence following a first unprovoked seizure: a quantitative review. Neurology 1991;41:965–72.
8. Hesdorffer DC, Benn EK, Cascino GD, et al. Is a first acute symptomatic seizure epilepsy? Mortality and risk for recurrent seizure. Epilepsia 2009;50:1102–8.
9. Kim LG, Johnson TL, Marson AG, et al. Prediction of risk of seizure recurrence after a single seizure and early epilepsy: further results from the MESS trial. Lancet Neurol 2006;5:317–22.
10. Krumholz A, Wiebe S, Gronseth GS, et al. Evidence-based guideline: management of an unprovoked first seizure in adults: report of the guideline development subcommittee of the American Academy of Neurology and the American Epilepsy Society. Neurology 2015;84:1705–13.
11. NICE. The epilepsies: the diagnosis and management of the epilepsies in adults and children in primary and secondary care. Manchester (United Kingdom): NICE; 2015.

12. Krumholz A, Wiebe S, Gronseth G, et al. Practice Parameter: evaluating an apparent unprovoked first seizure in adults (an evidence-based review): report of the Quality Standards Subcommittee of the American Academy of Neurology and the American Epilepsy Society. Neurology 2007;69:1996–2007.
13. Wiebe S, Jette N. Pharmacoresistance and the role of surgery in difficult to treat epilepsy. Nat Rev Neurol 2012;8:669–77.
14. Berg AT, Berkovic SF, Brodie MJ, et al. Revised terminology and concepts for organization of seizures and epilepsies: report of the ILAE Commission on Classification and Terminology, 2005-2009. Epilepsia 2010;51:676–85.
15. Falip M, Gil-Nagel A, Viteri Torres C, et al. Diagnostic problems in the initial assessment of epilepsy. Neurologist 2007;13:S2–10.
16. Heo JH, Kim DW, Lee SY, et al. Reliability of semiology description. Neurologist 2008;14:7–11.
17. Tellez-Zenteno JF, Patten SB, Jette N, et al. Psychiatric comorbidity in epilepsy: a population-based analysis. Epilepsia 2007;48:2336–44.
18. Baca CB, Vickrey BG, Caplan R, et al. Psychiatric and medical comorbidity and quality of life outcomes in childhood-onset epilepsy. Pediatrics 2011;128: e1532–1543.
19. Taylor RS, Sander JW, Taylor RJ, et al. Predictors of health-related quality of life and costs in adults with epilepsy: a systematic review. Epilepsia 2011;52: 2168–80.
20. Fiest KM, Patten SB, Altura KC, et al. Patterns and frequency of the treatment of depression in persons with epilepsy. Epilepsy Behav 2014;39:59–64.
21. Kerr MP, Mensah S, Besag F, et al. International consensus clinical practice statements for the treatment of neuropsychiatric conditions associated with epilepsy. Epilepsia 2011;52:2133–8.
22. Carreno M, Donaire A, Sanchez-Carpintero R. Cognitive disorders associated with epilepsy: diagnosis and treatment. Neurologist 2008;14:S26–34.
23. Hermann B, Seidenberg M, Jones J. The neurobehavioural comorbidities of epilepsy: can a natural history be developed? Lancet Neurol 2008;7:151–60.
24. Kwan P, Arzimanoglou A, Berg AT, et al. Definition of drug resistant epilepsy: consensus proposal by the ad hoc Task Force of the ILAE Commission on Therapeutic Strategies. Epilepsia 2010;51:1069–77.
25. Engel J Jr, Wiebe S, French J, et al. Practice parameter: temporal lobe and localized neocortical resections for epilepsy: report of the Quality Standards Subcommittee of the American Academy of Neurology, in association with the American Epilepsy Society and the American Association of Neurological Surgeons. Neurology 2003;60:538–47.
26. Labiner DM, Bagic AI, Herman ST, et al. Essential services, personnel, and facilities in specialized epilepsy centers–revised 2010 guidelines. Epilepsia 2010;51: 2322–33.
27. Cross JH, Jayakar P, Nordli D, et al. Proposed criteria for referral and evaluation of children for epilepsy surgery: recommendations of the Subcommission for Pediatric Epilepsy Surgery. Epilepsia 2006;47:952–9.
28. Wiebe S, Jette N. Epilepsy surgery utilization: who, when, where, and why? Curr Opin Neurol 2012;25:187–93.
29. Jette N, Quan H, Tellez-Zenteno JF, et al. Development of an online tool to determine appropriateness for an epilepsy surgery evaluation. Neurology 2012;79: 1084–93.
30. Roberts JI, Hrazdil C, Wiebe S, et al. Feasibility of using an online tool to assess appropriateness for an epilepsy surgery evaluation. Neurology 2014;83:913–9.

31. Engel J Jr, McDermott MP, Wiebe S, et al. Early surgical therapy for drug-resistant temporal lobe epilepsy: a randomized trial. JAMA 2012;307:922–30.
32. Helmstaedter C, Kurthen M, Lux S, et al. Chronic epilepsy and cognition: a longitudinal study in temporal lobe epilepsy. Ann Neurol 2003;54:425–32.

Screening for Depression and Anxiety in Epilepsy

Kirsten M. Fiest, PhD[a], Scott B. Patten, MD, PhD, FRCPC[b,c],
Nathalie Jetté, MD, MSc, FRCPC[d,e],*

KEYWORDS

- Depression • Anxiety • Epilepsy • Screening • Measurement

KEY POINTS

- Many tools exist to screen for depression in epilepsy, although only a few for anxiety have been developed.
- The definitive tool to screen for depression in epilepsy has yet to be established.
- There have been few studies validating screening tools for anxiety in persons with epilepsy.

INTRODUCTION

Depression and anxiety are common in persons with epilepsy. Psychiatric disorders can have negative effects on quality of life, employment, and other epilepsy-related outcomes (eg, seizure outcome). Despite the high prevalence of depression and anxiety in epilepsy, they remain under-recognized and improperly treated. To adequately

Disclosures: N. Jetté holds a Canada Research Chair in Neurological Health Services Research. The authors have no commercial or financial conflicts of interest.
[a] Department of Internal Medicine, Health Sciences Centre, College of Medicine, University of Manitoba, 820 Sherbrook Street, MS740B, Winnipeg, Manitoba R3A 1R9, Canada; [b] Department of Community Health Sciences, Foothills Medical Centre, Cumming School of Medicine, University of Calgary, 3rd Floor TRW Building, 3280 Hospital Drive Northwest, Calgary, Alberta T2N 4Z6, Canada; [c] Department of Psychiatry, Mathison Centre for Mental Health Research & Education, Foothills Medical Centre, Cumming School of Medicine, University of Calgary, 3rd Floor TRW Building, 3280 Hospital Drive Northwest, Calgary, Alberta T2N 4Z6, Canada; [d] Department of Clinical Neurosciences, Hotchkiss Brain Institute, Foothills Medical Centre, Cumming School of Medicine, University of Calgary, 1403 29 Street Northwest, Calgary, Alberta T2N 2T9, Canada; [e] Department of Community Health Sciences, O'Brien Institute for Public Health, Foothills Medical Centre, Cumming School of Medicine, University of Calgary, 1403 29 Street Northwest, Calgary, Alberta T2N 2T9, Canada
* Corresponding author. Department of Clinical Neurosciences, Hotchkiss Brain Institute, Foothills Medical Centre, Cumming School of Medicine, University of Calgary, 1403 29 Street Northwest, Calgary, Alberta T2N 2T9, Canada.
E-mail address: nathalie.jette@albertahealthservices.ca

Neurol Clin 34 (2016) 351–361
http://dx.doi.org/10.1016/j.ncl.2015.11.003
neurologic.theclinics.com

identify depression or anxiety in persons with epilepsy, screening tools are often recommended to ensure their rapid detection and appropriate management.

DEFINITION, EPIDEMIOLOGY, AND IMPACT OF DEPRESSION AND ANXIETY IN EPILEPSY

A major depressive episode (MDE) can be described as depressed mood and/or markedly diminished interest in almost all activities, accompanied by any number of physical or psychological symptoms (**Box 1**). At least 5 of 9 specified symptoms are required for a diagnosis of MDE, along with certain exclusion criteria, such as past manic episode (which indicates that an MDE was a manifestation of a bipolar disorder rather than a major depressive disorder [MDD]).[1] Common features of an MDE include fatigue, appetite changes, sleep changes, psychomotor agitation or retardation (restlessness or moving more slowly than normal), difficulties with concentration, feelings of worthlessness or guilt, and suicidal thoughts, plans, or attempts.[1] According to the *Diagnostic and Statistical Manual* (Fifth Edition) (*DSM-5*), symptoms must persist for at least 2 weeks and cause marked distress or interfere with social, occupational, or educational functioning to be considered an MDE.[1] MDD includes both single MDEs and recurrent depressive episodes, although it is distinguished from depressive symptoms, which alone do not indicate clinical depression. Based on the *DSM-5*, the hallmarks of a depressive disorder, as opposed to depressive symptoms, is that the clinically recognizable cluster of symptoms must be combined with distress, disability, or increased risk of death, pain, disability, or an important loss of freedom.[1] In distinction to this clinically defined syndrome, self-report rating scales assess depressive symptoms along a continuum of severity or dimension. The dimensional assessment of symptoms may be useful in screening applications but it is not equivalent to categorically defined MDE and MDD. The term depression is used in this article to describe a single MDE or recurrent MDEs and *depressive symptoms* is used to describe those characteristics that may indicate depression but on their own are not sufficient for diagnosis.

Box 1
***Diagnostic and Statistical Manual of Mental Disorders* diagnostic criteria for a major depressive episode**

Depressed mood and/or diminished interest or pleasure in life activities for at least 2 weeks and at least 5 of the following symptoms that cause clinically significant impairment in social, work, or other important areas of functioning almost every day:

Depressed mood most of the day

Loss of interest or pleasure in all or most activities

Significant unintentional weight loss or gain (or changes in appetite)

Insomnia or sleeping too much

Psychomotor agitation or retardation (noticed by others)

Fatigue or loss of energy

Feelings of worthlessness or excessive guilt

Diminished ability to think or concentrate, or indecisiveness

Recurrent thoughts of death

Note: MDD requires 2 or more MDEs.

Anxiety often refers to the body's natural warning response; it becomes pathologic when it is excessive and uncontrollable. Anxiety disorders are a broad group of syndromes, as previously outlined in the *Diagnostic and Statistical Manual of Mental Disorders* (Fourth Edition, Text Revision) (*DSM-IV-TR*),[2] including panic disorder, agoraphobia, social phobia, specific phobia, obsessive-compulsive disorder (OCD), posttraumatic stress disorder (PTSD), and generalized anxiety disorder (GAD). OCD and PTSD have been removed to separate chapters in the *DSM-5*, apart from other anxiety disorders.[1] Each anxiety disorder is defined by a distinct cluster of symptoms, present over varying periods of time, that cause a person significant distress or interfere with daily functioning.[1] A majority of tools to assess anxiety in research focus on GAD (**Box 2**), which is marked by chronic, irrational, and excessive worry about everyday life events and activity. Symptoms of GAD include irritability, muscle tension, restlessness, sleep disturbance, fatigue, and difficulty concentrating; these symptoms must occur more days than not for at least 6 months to meet the *Diagnostic and Statistical Manual of Mental Disorders (DSM)* criteria for GAD.[1,2]

In the general population, the lifetime prevalence of major depression is estimated to be 12% to 16%,[3–5] with a prevalence in the past year between 3.9% and 6.6%[3–5] and in the past 30 days of 1.8%.[3] Major depression is more common in women than in men, and the peak prevalence occurs between the ages of 15 and 25 years.[3] The prevalence of depression in epilepsy is markedly higher than in the general population; persons with epilepsy have 3 times the odds of depression relative to those without epilepsy.[6] Anxiety disorders are common in the general population, with lifetime prevalence estimates of specific phobia (18.4%), social phobia (13.0%), PTSD (10.1%), GAD (9.0%), and OCD (2.7%).[7] There is less research on anxiety disorders in persons with epilepsy, relative to depression. The lifetime prevalence of anxiety disorders in persons with epilepsy was 22.8% in a population-based study, with a 12-month prevalence of 12.8%.[8] Other studies have replicated these findings, reporting prevalence estimates of anxiety ranging between 15% and 27%.[9,10]

Depression and anxiety have a substantial impact on persons with epilepsy, affecting quality of life, seizure control, and use of the health care system and contribute to adverse effects of antiepileptic medication and other psychosocial problems.[11] Park and colleagues[12] reported that affective symptoms were most associated with quality of life, and those with poorly controlled seizures, in addition to affective symptoms, had the lowest quality of life. Interictal symptoms of depression and anxiety have been reported as the strongest predictors of quality of life, more

---

Box 2
Diagnostic and Statistical Manual of Mental Disorders **diagnostic criteria for generalized anxiety disorder**

The presence of excessive anxiety and worry about a variety of topics, events, or activities. Worry occurs more often than not for at least 6 months. The anxiety and worry are associated with at least 3 of the following physical or cognitive symptoms:

Edginess or restlessness

Tiring easily or being more fatigued than usual

Impaired concentration

Irritability

Increased muscle aches or soreness

Difficulty sleeping

so than the severity and frequency of seizures in 1 study.[13] Levels of felt stigma and suicidal ideation are highest in those with depression or anxiety.[9] Adverse events from antiepileptic drugs, including headache and memory problems, were enhanced in those with subthreshold symptoms of depression and anxiety.[14] Early identification and management of symptoms of depression and anxiety in persons with epilepsy may provide benefits above and beyond the relief of psychiatric symptoms.

MEASURING DEPRESSION AND ANXIETY

Depression and anxiety are diagnosed by many methods in practice, including structured and semistructured interviews, questionnaires (which are used as surrogates for diagnosis or as indicators for further assessment), and clinical judgment based on DSM-5 criteria. In most settings, however, in which formal measures are taken (eg, for screening) depressive symptom rating scales are used. Some of the most commonly used questionnaires in the general population are the Hospital Anxiety and Depression Scale (HADS),[15] the Patient Health Questionnaire (PHQ),[16] and the Generalized Anxiety Disorder 7-item scale (GAD-7).[17] Each of these methods varies in terms of adoption, feasibility, and accuracy.

SCREENING

The suitability of tools for the assessment of depression or anxiety in epilepsy can be judged in many ways. Given the existence of a suitable gold standard in the Structured Clinical Interview for DSM Disorders (SCID), measures of the accuracy of these instruments can include sensitivity, specificity, positive predictive value (PPV), negative predictive value (NPV), and area under the curve (AUC). These measures are useful in comparing measures within and between different groups of people. Several approaches exist to assess depression in epilepsy, each with their own strengths and weaknesses. The possibility for bias should always be considered when conducting assessments, and steps should be taken to mitigate the magnitude of this bias.

There is often ambiguity when discussing screening; there is the classic idea of secondary prevention, where the goal is to detect a disease in its early stages, before symptoms appear, and intervening to stop or slow its progression. In contrast, there may be depression and anxiety under the surface and the belief that it can be brought into awareness and action by detecting its presence – which is another interpretation of the concept. Often, self-report inventories for depression and anxiety are used in the context of screening in the latter interpretation. For screening to be effective, a tool must meet a certain number of criteria: (1) it should produce a better prognosis than if it were detected and treated later; (2) it should be inexpensive and quick; (3) it should not result in many false-positive results, which could result in inappropriate treatment, increased burden to the health care system, and the potential of being stigmatized and labeled; (4) it should be important and prevalent and cannot be easily detected without screening; and (5) there should be appropriate, available, and effective follow-up treatment.[18,19] If depression or anxiety are identified and treated sooner in persons with epilepsy, it is hypothesized there may be fewer or less severe psychosocial consequences, the risk of suicide may be decreased, and a degeneration of limbic structures may be slowed.[20,21] Several screening instruments for depression and anxiety in epilepsy are publically available at no cost and typically take less than 5 minutes to complete.[11,22] The high prevalence of depression and anxiety in epilepsy will lead to a decreased number of false-positive results. Depression and anxiety are difficult to diagnose quickly in a clinical setting without the use of a screening tool. Validated treatments for depression and anxiety exist in the general population, including most selective serotonin reuptake inhibitors (SSRIs) and therapy with an expert, such as a psychiatrist or clinical psychologist; they are viewed as effective in epilepsy, although this has not been tested in any large randomized controlled trials.[22,23] Taking this into account, screening for depression and anxiety in persons with epilepsy should be considered in clinical settings, potentially leading to an improved prognosis. The most recent recommendations, published by the International League Against Epilepsy Commission on the Neuropsychiatric Aspects of Epilepsy, recommend screening for depression in all new and existing cases of epilepsy with either the PHQ-2 or the Neurologic Disorders Depression Inventory for Epilepsy (NDDI-E).[22] These recommendations, however, preceded the publication of several important validation studies. Also, consensus groups have not, as yet, recommended screening instruments for anxiety.

TOOLS TO SCREEN FOR DEPRESSION AND ANXIETY IN EPILEPSY

Fully structured and semistructured interviews, such as the Composite International Diagnostic Interview (CIDI) and SCID, are rarely used in clinical settings and screening. The Mini-International Neuropsychiatric Interview (MINI) was designed for use by clinicians, although its structure may be inconvenient for use in practice. These formal interviews are more commonly used as the standard by which to assess the performance of screening instruments, such as self-reported rating scales. The metrics used to assess the accuracy of screening tools (ie, sensitivity and specificity) are used to judge how well an instrument performs relative to a gold standard measurement.[24] The values calculated by these measures are useful to determine the ability of different measurement approaches to correctly assess an outcome.[24] In the following examples, the utility of various approaches to assessing depression and anxiety in people with epilepsy is discussed in the context of these accuracy measures.

Structured Interviews

Composite International Diagnostic Interview

The CIDI was developed at the request of the World Health Organization and a branch of the United States government.[25] The CIDI is primarily intended for use in the general population and is widely used in international epidemiologic surveys. Forty *DSM* (Third Edition) disorders are covered in the CIDI, including single and recurrent episodes of major depression and several anxiety disorders.[25] Lifetime, past year, and current psychiatric disorders are probed. As a fully structured interview, the CIDI may be administered by trained laypersons; a computer makes diagnoses based on algorithms for those conditions covered.[25] The CIDI can be long, lasting approximately 1 hour (although the length of the interview is variable due to its branched structure), and the software and scoring system must be purchased.[25] The CIDI has a modular structure, so it can be used in a way that covers only 1 or a few disorders. The CIDI can be self-administered via a computer, suggesting it could be used for screening, but the length of the interview can be variable due to its branching logic, and it is rarely used in this way.

Mini-International Neuropsychiatric Interview

The MINI is a brief, structured clinical interview designed to assess psychiatric disorders in epidemiologic studies and clinical trials.[26] As its name suggests, the MINI is fast to administer, taking approximately 15 minutes.[26] The MINI was designed to be quick, inexpensive, highly sensitive, highly specific, and compatible with international diagnostic criteria, including the *International Classification of Diseases-10* and *DSM-IV*.[26]

The MINI mainly assesses current psychopathology, although a limited number of lifetime disorders are also probed for some conditions, such as panic and psychotic disorders.[26] Also, even though the MINI is brief, a 15-minute psychiatric interview is difficult to implement in busy neurologic clinics.

Semistructured Interviews

Structured Clinical Interview for DSM

The SCID is a semistructured assessment tool for psychiatric conditions, widely considered the gold standard in research.[27] As the name suggests, the SCID is based entirely on *DSM* criteria and includes sections for both current and lifetime depression and multiple anxiety disorders.[1] The SCID is a top-down assessment instrument; *DSM* criteria are the starting point and for depression a person must meet 5 of the 9 symptoms (1 of which must be depressed mood or anhedonia) to be classified as depressed.[27] Each anxiety disorder is assessed individually, with varying criteria; what they all have in common is the necessity for impairment in social, family, or occupational functioning. The semistructured format has its advantages; there is a degree of standardization, although it allows adequate flexibility in asking follow-up questions.[27] For research purposes, the SCID is available for free, as long as notification to the copyright holders has been given. A disadvantage is that laypersons cannot administer the SCID, because content knowledge is required to ask the appropriate follow-up questions.[27] The SCID is also more time consuming than self-report inventories, taking from 15 to 150 minutes to complete depending on the number of modules included and whether the respondent has psychiatric symptoms or not.

Self-Report

Several self-report methods exist to assess depression and anxiety in epilepsy; some are generic, whereas others are disease specific (**Table 1**).

Patient Health Questionnaire

The PHQ-9 is a 9-item self-report instrument used to assess depressive symptoms and can be used to establish a syndrome of depression that is likely to indicate major depression as well as establishing the severity of symptoms.[16] It can be scored either using an algorithm for the MDE or with a cutpoint-based interpretation of the total score. The PHQ-9 follows the *DSM-IV-TR* criteria with both the timing (past 2 weeks) and persistence (through item response choices) criteria. All 9 items are scored from

Table 1
Commonly used tools to screen for depression or anxiety in epilepsy

Tool	Abbreviation	Condition Assessed	Number of Items	Validated in Epilepsy	Publically Available
Patient Health Questionnaire[16]	PHQ	Depression	2/9	Yes[28,29]	Yes
Neurologic Disorders Depression Inventory for Epilepsy[30]	NDDI-E	Depression	6	Yes[30]	Yes
Hospital Anxiety and Depression Scale[15]	HADS	Depression and anxiety	7 For each subscale	Yes[28,37]	No
Generalized Anxiety Disorder 7-item scale[17]	GAD-7	Anxiety	7	Yes[11]	Yes

0 to 3: 0 indicates the problems did not bother the person at all and 3 that they bothered the person nearly every day. As a severity measure, scores of 0 to 4 indicate minimal/no depression, 5 to 9 mild depression, 10 to 14 moderate depression, 15 to 19 moderately severe depression, and 20 to 27 severe depression. The first 2 items of the PHQ-9 are in themselves considered a tool for assessing depression: the PHQ-2. The PHQ-2 includes only the 2 cardinal symptoms of depression, anhedonia and depressed mood—the endorsement of 1 of these symptoms more than half of the days in a 2-week period indicates the possibility of major depression.

The PHQ has been assessed as a screening tool in epilepsy in 2 studies.[28,29] Fiest and colleagues'[28] study validated all scoring methods of the PHQ: the PHQ-2, PHQ-9 cutpoint, and PHQ-9 algorithm. The PHQ-9 at a cutpoint of 9 had the best balance of sensitivity and specificity (AUC: 88%) and was deemed acceptable for use in those with epilepsy followed in a tertiary-care program. The PHQ-2 and PHQ-9 algorithm had suboptimal AUCs, although the specificity of the PHQ-9 algorithm had the highest specificity (96.2%) of all the tools tested. Rathore and colleagues'[29] study used the MINI to validate the PHQ-9 in 172 persons with epilepsy. At a cutpoint of 10, the estimated AUC was 91.4%, sensitivity 92.0%, and specificity 74.0%.

Critics of the PHQ-9 believe that the somatic symptoms of depression could overlap with common side effects of antiepileptic medications, invalidating its use in this population.[14] Decreased concentration, fatigue, and difficulties sleeping may be medication side effects that are also questions on the PHQ-9. Despite this, it seems a useful screening tool for depression in epilepsy, although further validation is needed.

Neurologic Disorders Depression Inventory for Epilepsy

The NDDI-E is a disease-specific depression assessment tool and was proposed as an alternative to general depression scales for use in epilepsy.[30] According to the study investigators, adverse antiepileptic drug effects and the cognitive symptoms of epilepsy do not confound the items of the NDDI-E.[21] For these reasons, it is viewed by the study group as the most acceptable tool for measuring depression in epilepsy. The scale contains 6 items (everything is a struggle; nothing I do is right; feel guilty; I'd be better off dead; frustrated; and difficulty finding pleasure) that are scored from 1 (never) to 4 (always or often). Scores of greater than 15 on the NDDI-E are suggestive of a diagnosis of depression.[30]

The utility of this scale has been assessed in many populations. In the original article,[7] the investigators validated the NDDI-E against a MINI diagnosis of depression. A diagnosis of depression was established in 17% of more than 200 adult outpatients with epilepsy; a PPV of 0.62, NPV of 0.96, sensitivity of 0.81, and specificity of 0.90 were found using the suggested 15-point cutoff. Margrove and colleagues[31] validated the NDDI-E against the MINI and found a PPV of 0.86, NPV of 1.0, sensitivity of 1.0, and specificity of 0.85 (with a prevalence of depression of 39.5%). A study of 266 persons with epilepsy by Rampling and colleagues[32] found a PPV of the NDDI-E of only 0.506 in a population with a prevalence of depression of 17.7%.

Although many studies have been conducted, the NDDI-E does not convincingly outperform general depression scales in terms of its validity in persons with epilepsy. Low PPVs are associated with a high number of false-positive results; resources may be diverted and treatment required for many persons who do not actually have depression.[24] In spite of these limitations, the scale is widely available, free, and takes only 3 minutes to complete, and several translations of the scale (eg, Brazilian-Portuguese, German, Italian, and Japanese) have also been validated.[33–36] More research is required to directly compare these general and disease-specific means of assessing depression in persons with epilepsy.

Hospital Anxiety and Depression Scale

The HADS is a brief, self-report inventory for assessing symptoms of both depression (HADS-D) and anxiety (HADS-A).[15] The depressive symptoms of the HADS-D are different from most scales, because they do not map directly onto *DSM* criteria. The depression items include, "I can laugh and see the funny side of things," "I feel cheerful," and "I have lost interest in my appearance." The anxiety items of the HADS-A include, "I feel tense or 'wound up'," "Worrying thoughts go through my mind," and "I can sit at ease and feel relaxed." Each item is scored from 0 to 3, although the response choices differ for each question.

The recommended cutoff for the depression subscale of the HADS-D in persons with epilepsy is 7 of 13.[28,37] When validated against scores on the CIDI, a score of 7 yielded a sensitivity of 0.909 and a specificity of 1.0.[37] At these cutoffs the HADS-D seems a useful screening instrument for depression in persons with epilepsy. Two studies have assessed the use of the HADS-A as a screening tool for anxiety in persons with epilepsy.[31,38] The first study validating the HADS-A in epilepsy reported high sensitivities (83%–91%) and specificities (85%–94%) when using a cutpoint of 7 or 8 compared with the CIDI.[37] In an article by Gandy and colleagues,[38] the investigators deemed the HADS-A an inadequate measure for screening for anxiety disorders in epilepsy, because it had a low AUC (0.68) and poor sensitivity (61%) compared with a MINI diagnosis of anxiety. The specificity of the HADS for anxiety was deemed reasonable but overall inappropriate for screening (75%).

The HADS-D was specifically designed for use in patients with medical conditions and may have advantages over other general depression scales,[15] because it does not include somatic symptoms of depression that may also be side-effects of antiepileptic medication or the epilepsy disease process. One major downside of the HADS is its cost; it is not freely available and a license must be obtained for its use.

Generalized Anxiety Disorder-7

The GAD-7 is a brief clinical tool to assess symptoms of GAD, based on *DSM* criteria, along with symptoms commonly assessed in other anxiety measures.[17] Questions on the GAD-7 include, "having trouble relaxing," "not being able to stop or control worrying," and "becoming easily annoyed or irritable," with response choices ranging from not being bothered at all to being bothered nearly every day.[17] When validated against the GAD section of the SCID, the GAD-7 at a cutpoint of 10 resulted in optimal sensitivity (89%) and specificity (82%).[17] In persons with epilepsy, the GAD-7 has been validated against the MINI - Plus version 5.0.0.[11] In epilepsy, the optimal cutpoint for scoring the GAD-7 was 6, which resulted in a sensitivity of 92.2% and specificity of 89.1%—values higher than the original validation of this tool.[11] The GAD-7 correlated well with measures of depression, quality of life, and adverse medication effects in persons with epilepsy.[11] In addition to its validity in epilepsy, the GAD-7 is free to use and relatively brief.

SELECTING THE APPROPRIATE TOOL

The optimal tool for screening depends on many different factors, including the goals of screening (eg, research vs clinical applications), length, and cost. If the goal of a study were to identify depressed or anxious people, then high sensitivity would be required. If strong PPV were a key requirement, high specificity would be important. In a resource-scarce environment where the goal is to minimize false-positive results, the tool with the highest specificity may be preferred. If the intention of screening is to detect people who may be struggling with anxiety or depression – and to trigger early detection or draw attention to specific problems – then a lower level of performance may be sufficient, whereas if the goal is to detect people in need of psychiatric consultation for treatment of disorders, then a different, higher, standard might apply. Although depression and anxiety often are untreated in those with epilepsy, they are also often poorly managed[39]; screening might help detect people who need reassessment.

CONSIDERATIONS/KNOWLEDGE GAPS

There are important factors that must be carefully considered when discussing screening for psychiatric disorders in epilepsy. The first is that GAD is the only anxiety disorder measured in screening tools, although this is not an issue specific to epilepsy, because these tools are also used in other populations. The GAD-7 has a reputation of being able to detect a variety of disorders characterized by heightened anxiety, but validation studies are needed to further clarify its performance. Anxiety in epilepsy is understudied, relative to depression; this is especially true regarding the validity of anxiety screening tools in this population. In addition, the potential confounding influence of adverse antiepileptic drug side effects on the performance of both depression and anxiety screening tools must be considered.

SUMMARY

There is little evidence (eg, randomized controlled trials) to support the idea that formal screening improves outcomes in those with epilepsy, but it makes intuitive sense as highlighted in consensus statements. A formalized screening procedure, however, requires administrative support and a protocol for screen positive results, as noted by Thombs and colleagues,[19] and as such can be expensive and cumbersome. Less formal self-report screening instruments may help clinicians remain vigilant about determinants of quality of life that they may not otherwise think about, such as depression and anxiety, and that patients may not raise spontaneously, opening a door to constructive clinical actions. The implementation strategy of screening tools in different settings will depend on any initiative's needs and goals, the time available to clinicians, the mental health resources available, and the characteristics of the clientele.

Rating scales can be broadly split into 2 groups: those that provide dimensional scores and those that are categorical in nature. Dimensional scales (HADS and NDDI-E) give a person a number rather than a nominal categorization, and the arbitrary nature of categories, where information may be lost, is not a concern for some applications (such as identifying those in need of additional assessment). Categories (SCID and MINI) are also useful; nominal information is important for guideline treatment and can lead to meaningful action in terms of clinical need. One scale does exist that blends the 2: the PHQ-9 is a hybrid assessment tool that provides both dimensional and categorical information. Although much research has been conducted and the PHQ-9 and the NIDDI-E hold great promise for depression screening in epilepsy, the ideal tool for measuring depression in persons with epilepsy remains to be determined. Adequate validation of multiple depression screening questionnaires has not been conducted using the appropriate gold standard in a well-described, large population. There are also few studies assessing screening tools for anxiety in epilepsy. Future research should focus on validating multiple depression scales in the same sample and more anxiety inventories in persons with epilepsy to maximize the utility and benefit of these tools and generate more evidence-based research in the field.

REFERENCES

1. American Psychiatric Association. Diagnostic and statistical manual for mental disorders-5. Arlington (VA): American Psychiatric Publishing; 2013.
2. American Psychiatric Association. Diagnostic and statistical manual for mental disorders-IV-TR. Arlington (VA): American Psychiatric Publishing; 1994.
3. Patten SB, Wang JL, Williams JV, et al. Descriptive epidemiology of major depression in Canada. Can J Psychiatry 2006;51:84–90.
4. Kessler RC, Berglund P, Demler O, et al. The epidemiology of major depressive disorder: results from the National Comorbidity Survey Replication (NCS-R). JAMA 2003;289:3095–105.
5. Alonso J, Angermeyer MC, Bernert S, et al. Prevalence of mental disorders in Europe: results from the European Study of the Epidemiology of Mental Disorders (ESEMeD) project. Acta Psychiatr Scand Suppl 2004;(420):21–7.
6. Fiest KM, Dykeman J, Patten SB, et al. Depression in epilepsy: a systematic review and meta-analysis. Neurology 2013;80:590–9.
7. Kessler RC, Petukhova M, Sampson NA, et al. Twelve-month and lifetime prevalence and lifetime morbid risk of anxiety and mood disorders in the United States. Int J Methods Psychiatr Res 2012;21:169–84.
8. Tellez-Zenteno JF, Patten SB, Jette N, et al. Psychiatric comorbidity in epilepsy: a population-based analysis. Epilepsia 2007;48:2336–44.
9. Kwon OY, Park SP. Frequency of affective symptoms and their psychosocial impact in Korean people with epilepsy: a survey at two tertiary care hospitals. Epilepsy Behav 2013;26:51–6.
10. Fiest KM, Wiebe S, Patten S, et al. Symptoms of anxiety in persons with epilepsy. 31st International Epilepsy Congress. Istanbul, Turkey, September 2015.
11. Seo JG, Cho YW, Lee SJ, et al. Validation of the generalized anxiety disorder-7 in people with epilepsy: a MEPSY study. Epilepsy Behav 2014;35:59–63.
12. Park SP, Song HS, Hwang YH, et al. Differential effects of seizure control and affective symptoms on quality of life in people with epilepsy. Epilepsy Behav 2010; 18:455–9.
13. Johnson EK, Jones JE, Seidenberg M, et al. The relative impact of anxiety, depression, and clinical seizure features on health-related quality of life in epilepsy. Epilepsia 2004;45:544–50.
14. Kanner AM, Barry JJ, Gilliam F, et al. Depressive and anxiety disorders in epilepsy: do they differ in their potential to worsen common antiepileptic drug-related adverse events? Epilepsia 2012;53:1104–8.
15. Zigmond AS, Snaith RP. The hospital anxiety and depression scale. Acta Psychiatr Scand 1983;67:361–70.
16. Kroenke K, Spitzer RL, Williams JB. The PHQ-9: validity of a brief depression severity measure. J Gen Intern Med 2001;16:606–13.
17. Spitzer RL, Kroenke K, Williams JB, et al. A brief measure for assessing generalized anxiety disorder: the GAD-7. Arch Intern Med 2006;166:1092–7.
18. Mitchell AJ. Clinical utility of screening for clinical depression and bipolar disorder. Curr Opin Psychiatry 2012;25:24–31.
19. Thombs BD, Coyne JC, Cuijpers P, et al. Rethinking recommendations for screening for depression in primary care. CMAJ 2012;184:413–8.
20. Kanner AM. Depression in epilepsy: a neurobiologic perspective. Epilepsy Curr 2005;5:21–7.
21. Kanner AM. Depression and epilepsy: a review of multiple facets of their close relation. Neurol Clin 2009;27:865–80.

22. Kerr MP, Mensah S, Besag F, et al. International consensus clinical practice statements for the treatment of neuropsychiatric conditions associated with epilepsy. Epilepsia 2011;52:2133–8.
23. Schmitz B. Antidepressant drugs: indications and guidelines for use in epilepsy. Epilepsia 2002;43(Suppl 2):14–8.
24. Oleckno WA. Epidemiology: concepts and methods. Long Grove (IL): Waveland Press, Inc; 2008.
25. Robins LN, Wing J, Wittchen HU, et al. The Composite International Diagnostic Interview. An epidemiologic Instrument suitable for use in conjunction with different diagnostic systems and in different cultures. Arch Gen Psychiatry 1988;45:1069–77.
26. Sheehan DV, Lecrubier Y, Sheehan KH, et al. The Mini-International Neuropsychiatric Interview (M.I.N.I.): the development and validation of a structured diagnostic psychiatric interview for DSM-IV and ICD-10. J Clin Psychiatry 1998; 59(Suppl 20):22–33 [quiz: 34–57].
27. Sanchez-Villegas A, Schlatter J, Ortuno F, et al. Validity of a self-reported diagnosis of depression among participants in a cohort study using the Structured Clinical Interview for DSM-IV (SCID-I). BMC Psychiatry 2008;8:43.
28. Fiest KM, Patten SB, Wiebe S, et al. Validating screening tools for depression in epilepsy. Epilepsia 2014;55:1642–50.
29. Rathore JS, Jehi LE, Fan Y, et al. Validation of the Patient Health Questionnaire-9 (PHQ-9) for depression screening in adults with epilepsy. Epilepsy Behav 2014; 37:215–20.
30. Gilliam FG, Barry JJ, Hermann BP, et al. Rapid detection of major depression in epilepsy: a multicentre study. Lancet Neurol 2006;5:399–405.
31. Margrove K, Mensah S, Thapar A, et al. Depression screening for patients with epilepsy in a primary care setting using the Patient Health Questionnaire-2 and the neurological disorders depression inventory for epilepsy. Epilepsy Behav 2011;21:387–90.
32. Rampling J, Mitchell AJ, Von Oertzen T, et al. Screening for depression in epilepsy clinics. A comparison of conventional and visual-analog methods. Epilepsia 2012;53:1713–21.
33. de Oliveira GN, Kummer A, Salgado JV, et al. Brazilian version of the Neurological Disorders Depression Inventory for Epilepsy (NDDI-E). Epilepsy Behav 2010;19:328–31.
34. Mula M, Iudice A, La Neve A, et al. Validation of the Italian version of the Neurological Disorders Depression Inventory for Epilepsy (NDDI-E). Epilepsy Behav 2012;24:329–31.
35. Metternich B, Wagner K, Buschmann F, et al. Validation of a German version of the Neurological Disorders Depression Inventory for Epilepsy (NDDI-E). Epilepsy Behav 2012;25:485–8.
36. Tadokoro Y, Oshima T, Fukuchi T, et al. Screening for major depressive episodes in Japanese patients with epilepsy: validation and translation of the Japanese version of Neurological Disorders Depression Inventory for Epilepsy (NDDI-E). Epilepsy Behav 2012;25:18–22.
37. Al-Asmi A, Dorvlo AS, Burke DT, et al. The detection of mood and anxiety in people with epilepsy using two-phase designs: experiences from a tertiary care centre in Oman. Epilepsy Res 2012;98:174–81.
38. Gandy M, Sharpe L, Perry KN, et al. Anxiety in epilepsy: a neglected disorder. J Psychosom Res 2015;78:149–55.
39. Fiest KM, Patten SB, Altura KC, et al. Patterns and frequency of the treatment of depression in persons with epilepsy. Epilepsy Behav 2014;39:59–64.

Starting, Choosing, Changing, and Discontinuing Drug Treatment for Epilepsy Patients

CrossMark

Dieter Schmidt, MD

KEYWORDS

- Antiepileptic drugs • Epilepsy drug therapy • Starting antiepileptic drugs
- Stopping antiepileptic drugs • Optimizing antiepileptic drugs

KEY POINTS

- Antiepileptic drug (AED) therapy should be offered as soon as epilepsy has been established.
- In new-onset epilepsy, 80% of patients will enter lasting seizure remission during drug therapy.
- AED therapy needs to be changed in those with poor seizure control, relevant side effects, or both.
- Stopping AEDs is most successful in those entering remission early and with no history of prior withdrawal attempts.

Epilepsy is a serious brain disease encompassing many different seizure types and epilepsy syndromes, some of which are life-shortening.[1] Fortunately, up to 80% of patients with new-onset epilepsy have complete seizure control with current antiepileptic drug (AED) therapy,[2,3] and 60% remain seizure free even after AEDs have been withdrawn.[4] This outcome makes epilepsy one of the best treatable chronic brain diseases if AEDs are used optimally, which includes knowing how to start, how to change, and how to stop AEDs. In this article, the current drug therapy of epilepsy in adults is briefly reviewed. Treatment of special treatment groups, such as women and children, those with comorbidities, emergency care, and nonpharmacological treatments, is beyond the scope of this short article and is covered elsewhere in this issue.

Disclosure Statement: The author has received honoraria for speaker and consultant services in the last 2 years from Eisai, Medichem, Novartis, Shire, Sun Pharma, UCB, and Viropharm.
Epilepsy Research Group, Goethestr.5, Berlin D-14163, Germany
E-mail address: dbschmidt@t-online.de

Neurol Clin 34 (2016) 363–381
http://dx.doi.org/10.1016/j.ncl.2015.11.007

WHY AND WHEN TO START THE FIRST ANTIEPILEPTIC DRUG?

Starting an AED, which is better called an antiseizure drug, after a first seizure reduces, if it works, the risk of a second seizure compared with no or delayed treatment.[5] Whether some AEDs have the ability to change the underlying disease beyond symptomatic seizure control is under discussion but is beyond the scope of this article (see Ref.[6]). Factors that put patients at high risk for seizure recurrence mainly include having a neurologic deficit or a brain lesion on MRI, having an abnormal electroencephalogram (EEG), and having a high frequency of seizures before starting treatment.[5] Recommending AED therapy after the first seizure is thus justifiable in patients at higher recurrence risk because high-risk patients have a slightly better long-term outcome with early versus delayed treatment.[5] Accordingly, the new, conceptual definition of epilepsy proposed by the International League Against Epilepsy (ILAE) includes patients after their first seizure if they carry a high risk of recurrent seizures.[7] One downside of the wider definition of epilepsy is that it extends the boundaries of epilepsy. Suddenly, more people have epilepsy than before and more people may be treated with AEDs than before when 2 seizures were commonly needed to diagnose epilepsy and to start AEDs. On the plus side, patients receive earlier treatment and may be spared from having further seizures.

For patients presenting with a history of 2 or more unprovoked seizures, which is still a commonly accepted clinical definition of epilepsy,[7] therapy with an AED is usually recommended, especially if further seizures carry the possibility of significant morbidity or mortality. This official ILAE recommendation is based on the influential clinical observation of a 73% risk of seizure recurrence within 4 years for those with a history of 2 prior unprovoked seizures.[8] The risk of a third seizure is nearly 2-fold higher in patients with remote symptomatic epilepsy than in those with genetic or no known cause.[8] Critics have noted that there are no randomized controlled trials in an unselected population of patients following 2 or more seizures to support this longstanding tradition and that the size of the treatment effect of AEDs is unclear.[9] If the diagnosis of epilepsy is uncertain, it is prudent not to initiate AED therapy but rather proceed to further evaluations, such as EEG monitoring, or adopt a watch-and-wait approach, at the discretion of the patient.[10]

Selecting the First Antiepileptic Drug

Ideally, AEDs used for the treatment of epilepsy should fully control seizures, be well tolerated with no long-term safety issues (such as teratogenicity, hypersensitivity reactions, or organ toxicity), and be easy to prescribe and take (once- or twice-daily dosage, no drug interactions, and no need for serum monitoring).[11] The introduction of 25 AEDs since the 1980s has offered more choices but has made the selection of the best suited drug for the individual patient perhaps more difficult, even for epilepsy specialists, because no available AED is ideal, and each has its advantages and limitations (**Table 1**). It is thought that prescribing a new drug is based entirely on a rational assessment of the scientific pros and cons of the agent, as presented in **Table 1**. However, recent research has uncovered that other factors may be more important. Suggestions by a pharmaceutical representative, observation of hospital prescribing, and a patient's request for a specific drug may play an important role.[24] Marketing efforts using recent insights from neuroeconomics that aim to appeal to the reward system in the mesial frontal lobe may possibly better explain why new AEDs are preferred, which seem to offer no substantial medical benefits over older drugs. In line with this observation, the

Table 1
Characteristics of widely used antiepileptic drugs for the treatment of epilepsy

AED[a]	Presumed Main Mechanism of Action	Approved Use (FDA, EMA)	Main Utility	Main Limitations
First generation				
Potassium bromide (1857)	GABA potentiation?	Generalized tonic–clonic seizures, myoclonic seizures	Use for focal and generalized seizures	Currently for adjunctive use only, not in wide use anymore, sedative
Phenobarbital (1912)	GABA potentiation	Partial and generalized convulsive seizures, sedation, anxiety disorders, sleep disorders	Use for focal and generalized seizures, IV use, the most cost-effective intervention for managing epilepsy, particularly for low-resource countries	Enzyme inducer, not useful in absence of seizures, skin hypersensitivity. Less effective than carbamazepine or phenytoin for focal seizures in mostly new-onset epilepsy[12]
Phenytoin (1938)	Na$^+$ channel blocker	Partial and generalized convulsive seizures	First-line AED, IV use, use for focal and generalized seizures with focal onset, first line AED, IV use, similar efficacy as carbamazepine[12]	Enzyme inducer, nonlinear pharmacokinetics, not useful for absence or myoclonic seizures, skin hypersensitivity
Primidone (1954)	GABA potentiation	Partial and generalized convulsive seizures	Use for focal and generalized seizures	Enzyme inducer, not useful for absence seizures, sedative, skin hypersensitivity. Less effective than carbamazepine or phenytoin for focal seizures in mostly new-onset epilepsy[12]
Ethosuximide (1958)	T-type Ca^{2+} channel blocker	Absence seizures	First-line AED, no skin hypersensitivity, use for absence seizures only; as effective as valproate for new-onset absence seizures[13]	Gastrointestinal side effects, insomnia, psychotic episodes

(continued on next page)

Table 1
(*continued*)

AED[a]	Presumed Main Mechanism of Action	Approved Use (FDA, EMA)	Main Utility	Main Limitations
Second generation				
Diazepam (1963)	GABA potentiation	Convulsive disorders, status epilepticus, anxiety, alcohol withdrawal	IV use, no clinical hepatotoxicity, no skin hypersensitivity, use for focal and generalized seizures	Currently for adjunctive use only, emergency use only, sedative, substantial tolerance (loss of efficacy)
Carbamazepine (1964)	Na$^+$ channel blockade	Partial and generalized convulsive seizures, trigeminal neuralgia, bipolar disorder	First-line AED, use for focal and generalized seizures with focal onset; none of the newer AEDs has currently been shown to be more efficacious than carbamazepine[14,15]	Enzyme inducer, not useful for absence or myoclonic seizures, skin hypersensitivity
Valproate (1967)	Multiple (eg., GABA potentiation, glutamate [NMDA] inhibition, sodium channel and T-type calcium channel blockade)	Partial and generalized convulsive seizures, absence seizures, migraine prophylaxis, bipolar disorder	First-line AED, IV use, no skin hypersensitivity, use for focal and generalized seizures; none of the newer AEDs has currently been shown to be more efficacious than valproate[15]	Enzyme inhibitor, substantial teratogenicity, weight gain
Clonazepam (1968)	GABA potentiation	Lennox–Gastaut syndrome, myoclonic seizures, panic disorders	No clinical hepatotoxicity, use for focal and generalized seizures	Currently for adjunctive use only, sedative, substantial tolerance (loss of efficacy)
Clobazam (1975)	GABA potentiation	Lennox–Gastaut syndrome, anxiety disorders	No clinical hepatotoxicity, use for focal and generalized seizures	Currently for adjunctive use only, sedative, substantial tolerance (loss of efficacy)

Third generation

Drug	Mechanism	Indications	Clinical use	Comments
Vigabatrin (1989)	GABA potentiation	Infantile spasms, complex partial seizures (currently for adjunctive use only)	No clinical hepatotoxicity, use for infantile spasms, focal and generalized seizures with focal onset	Not useful for absence or myoclonic seizures, visual field defect, weight gain; not as efficacious as carbamazepine for focal seizures[16]
Lamotrigine (1990)	Na+ channel blocker	Partial and generalized convulsive seizures, Lennox–Gastaut syndrome, bipolar disorder	First-line AED, use for focal and generalized seizures	Enzyme inducer, skin hypersensitivity, not as effective as valproate for new-onset absence seizures[13]
Oxcarbazepine (1990)	Na+ channel blocker	Partial seizures	First-line AED, use for focal and generalized seizures with focal onset	Enzyme inducer, hyponatremia, not useful for absence or myoclonic seizures, skin hypersensitivity
Gabapentin (1993)	Ca2+ blocker (α2δ subunit)	Partial and generalized convulsive seizures postherpetic and diabetic neuralgia, restless legs syndrome	No clinical hepatotoxicity, use for focal and generalized seizures with focal onset	Currently for adjunctive use only, not useful for absence or myoclonic seizures, weight gain. Not as effective as carbamazepine for new-onset focal seizures[17]
Topiramate (1995)	Multiple (GABA potentiation, glutamate [AMPA] inhibition, sodium and calcium channel blockade)	Partial and generalized convulsive seizures, Lennox–Gastaut syndrome, migraine prophylaxis	First-line AED, no clinical hepatotoxicity, use for focal and generalized seizures	Cognitive side effects, kidney stones, speech problems, weight loss. Not as effective as carbamazepine for new-onset focal seizures[17]
Levetiracetam (2000)	SV2A modulation	Partial and generalized convulsive seizures, partial seizures, generalized tonic–clonic seizures, juvenile myoclonic epilepsy	First-line AED, IV use, no clinical hepatotoxicity, use for focal and generalized seizures with focal onset and myoclonic seizures. As efficacious as carbamazepine for new-onset focal seizures[10]	Not useful for absence or myoclonic seizures, psychiatric side effects

(continued on next page)

Table 1
(continued)

AED[a]	Presumed Main Mechanism of Action	Approved Use (FDA, EMA)	Main Utility	Main Limitations
Zonisamide (2000)	Na$^+$ channel blocker	Partial seizures	First-line AED for focal seizures, no clinical hepatotoxicity, use for focal and generalized seizures; noninferior to carbamazepine for new-onset focal seizures[18]	Cognitive side effects, kidney stones, sedative, weight loss
Stiripentol (2002)	GABA potentiation, Na$^+$ channel blocker	Dravet syndrome	No clinical hepatotoxicity, use for seizures in Dravet syndrome	Currently for adjunctive use only
Pregabalin (2004)	Ca^{2+} blocker ($\alpha2\delta$ subunit)	Partial seizures, neuropathic pain, generalized anxiety disorder, fibromyalgia	No clinical hepatotoxicity, use for focal and generalized seizures with focal onset	Currently for adjunctive use only, not useful for absence or myoclonic seizures, weight gain
Rufinamide (2004)	Na$^+$ channel blockade	Lennox–Gastaut syndrome	No clinical hepatotoxicity, use for seizures in Lennox-Gastaut syndrome	Currently for adjunctive use only
Lacosamide (2008)	Enhanced slow inactivation of voltage-gated Na$^+$ channels	Partial seizures	No clinical hepatotoxicity, IV use, use for focal and generalized seizures with focal onset	Currently for adjunctive use only
Eslicarbazepine acetate (2009)	Na$^+$ channel blocker	Partial seizures	Use for focal and generalized seizures with focal onset	Currently for adjunctive use only, enzyme inducer, hyponatremia
Perampanel (2012)	Glutamate (AMPA) antagonist	Partial seizures	Use for focal and generalized seizures with focal onset	Currently for adjunctive use only, not useful for absence or myoclonic seizures

For details and less often used AEDs, see Refs.[19–23]

Abbreviations: AMPA, α-amino-3-hydroxy-5-methyl-4-isoxazolepropionic acid subtype of glutamate receptors; EMA, European Medicines Agency; FDA, US Food and Drug Administration; GABA, γ-aminobutyric acid; IV, intravenous; NMDA, N-methyl-D-aspartate subtype of glutamate receptors.

[a] Year in which the drug was first approved or marketed in the United States or Europe.

Adapted from Schmidt D, Schachter SC. Drug treatment of epilepsy in adults. BMJ 2014;348:g2546; with permission.

prescription of new drugs seems to be poorly affected by evidence for an added medical benefit or its absence,[25] suggesting that what drives physicians to prescribe a new AED beyond taking stock of the medical risk-benefit profile must be explored much better.

Treatment Effects of Antiepileptic Drugs in New-Onset Epilepsy

Most patients with newly diagnosed epilepsy undergoing AED therapy have a constant course, which can usually be predicted early.[26,27] As many as 50% of patients with new-onset focal or generalized seizures, as internationally defined,[28] become seizure-free while taking the first appropriately selected and dosed first-line AED.[27] The evidence base that a first-line AED is better than what is currently used is surprisingly limited to very few class I trials (**Table 2**, see Ref.[6] for review). The differences

---

Table 2
Preferred first-line antiepileptic drugs for new-onset and refractory epilepsy in adults

New-Onset Partial Epilepsies	Refractory Partial Epilepsies
Carbamazepine	Lacosamide
Gabapentin	Pregabalin
Lamotrigine	Zonisamide
Levetiracetam	Perampanel
Oxcarbazepine	Clobazam
Topiramate	
Valproate	

New-Onset Idiopathic Generalized Epilepsies	Refractory Idiopathic Generalized Epilepsies
Lamotrigine	Clobazam
Topiramate	Levetiracetam
Valproate	

This table takes into consideration the available class 1 evidence base for comparative efficacy and effectiveness in new-onset epilepsy, which is very sparse.[15,16] Uses approved by FDA and EMA (see **Table 3**). For refractory cases, all first-line AEDs for new-onset cases are also considered unless they have failed during previous treatment. For treatment of refractory partial epilepsy, pooled estimates of odds ratios (ORs) and number needed treat (NNT)/harm taking into account baseline risk were derived by random-effects meta-analysis.[29] Sixty-two placebo-controlled (12,902 patients) and 8 head-to-head randomized controlled trials (1370 patients) were included. Pooled ORs for responder and withdrawal rates (vs placebo) were 3.00 (95% confidence interval 2.63–3.41) and 1.48 (1.30–1.68), respectively. Indirect comparisons of responder rate based on relative measurements of treatment effect (ORs) favored topiramate (1.52; 1.06–2.20) in comparison with all other AEDs, whereas gabapentin (0.67; 0.46–0.97) and lacosamide (0.66; 0.48–0.92) were less efficacious, without significant heterogeneity. When analyses were based on absolute estimates (NNTs), topiramate and levetiracetam were more efficacious, whereas gabapentin and tiagabine were less efficacious. Withdrawal rate was higher with oxcarbazepine (OR 1.60; 1.12–2.29) and topiramate (OR 1.68; 1.07–2.63), and lower with gabapentin (OR 0.65; 0.42–1.00) and levetiracetam (OR 0.62; 0.43–0.89). The investigators conceded, however, that the differences found are of relatively small magnitude to allow a definitive conclusion about which new AED(s) has superior effectiveness. The author fully agrees with Costa and colleagues,[29] that the process of choosing AEDs for refractory partial epilepsy probably depends more on other aspects, such as individual patient characteristics and pharmacoeconomics, than on available controlled randomized evidence.

Data from Schmidt D, Schachter SC. Drug treatment of epilepsy in adults. BMJ 2014;348:g2546; and Löscher W, Schmidt D. Experimental and clinical evidence for loss of effect (tolerance) during prolonged treatment with antiepileptic drugs. Epilepsia 2006;47:1253–84; and *Modified from* Schmidt D. Drug treatment of epilepsy: options and limitations. Epilepsy Behav 2009;15:56–65; and Perucca, Tomson. The pharmacological treatment of epilepsy in adults. Lancet Neurol 2011;10(5):446-56.

Table 3
Overview of adverse effects of individual antiepileptic drugs

	CBZ	CLB	ESL	ETS	FBM	GBP	LCM	LEV	LTG	OXC	PGN	PER	PHB	PHT	TGB	RTG	TPM	VPA	VGB	ZNS
Early onset adverse events																				
Somnolence	−	++	+	+	−	+	+	+	+	−	+	−	++	−	++	+	++	−	+	++
Dizziness	−	++	−	+	−	+	+	+	+	++	−	−	−	++	++	−	++	−	+	+
Seizure aggravation	+	+	+	−	−	+	−	−	−	−	+	−	−	+	+	−	−	−	++	−
Gastrointestinal	+	−	−	++	(+)	(+)	−	(+)	−	+	−	−	−	−	−	−	−	+	−	+
Hypersensitivity (SJS/TEN)	+	−	+	+	+	−	−	−	+	+	−	−	+	+	−	−	+	−	−	+
Rash	+	−	−	−	−	−	−	−	+	+	−	−	+	+	−	−	−	−	−	−
Late onset adverse events																				
Encephalopathy	−	−	−	−	−	−	−	−	−	−	−	−	−	+	−	−	−	+	++	−
Depression	−	−	−	+	−	−	−	−	−	−	−	−	+	+	+	−	−	−	+	−
Behavioral problems	−	−	−	−	−	+	−	+	−	−	−	+	++	+	+	−	++	−	++	+
Psychotic episodes	(+)	−	−	++	(+)	+	−	(+)	−	−	−	−	(+)	(+)	(+)	−	(+)	(+)	++	−
Leucopenia	++	−	−	+	+	−	−	−	−	(+)	−	−	+	+	−	−	−	−	−	−
Aplastic anemia	+	−	−	+	++	−	−	−	−	−	−	−	+	+	−	−	−	−	−	−
Thrombocytopenia	−	−	−	−	+	−	−	−	−	−	−	−	−	−	−	−	−	++	−	−

Megaloblastic anemia

Pancreatitis

Liver failure

Nephrolithiasis

Osteoporosis

Hyponatremia

Weight gain

Weight loss

Cognition impaired

Teratogenicity

Retinal dysfunction

In general, the adverse effect profile of AEDs approved since 1985 appears to be advantageous compared with some of the classic AEDs (see summary of risks). It should be noted, however, that the incidence of many early-onset adverse events shown here could be lowered by slow titration, and avoiding above average dosages and combination therapy, if possible.

Abbreviations: +, risk higher than for AEDs without + sign; ++, highest risk among AEDs; AEDs, see **Table 1**; +, denotes minimally increased risk in clinical use.

Adapted from Löscher W, Klitgaard H, Twyman RE, et al. New avenues for anti-epileptic drug discovery and development. Nat Rev Drug Discov 2013;12(10):757–76; with permission; and *Modified from* Schmidt D. Drug treatment of epilepsy: options and limitations. Epilepsy Behav 2009;15:56–65; and Abou-Khalil B, Schmidt D. Antiepileptic drugs: advantages and disadvantages. In: Stefan H, Theodore WH, editors. Handbook of clinical neurology, vol. 108. Epilepsy part II: treatment. Amsterdam: Elsevier; 2012. p. 723–39.

are usually too small, if any, to allow a definitive conclusion about which new AEDs have superior effectiveness.[29] It was suggested that the process of choosing AEDs for refractory partial epilepsy probably depends more on other aspects, such as individual patient characteristics and pharmacoeconomics including marketing efforts, than on available controlled randomized evidence.[29] **Table 2** lists recommended AEDs for treatment of epilepsy in adults (see **Table 2**).

For example, a large unblinded but randomized study of AED monotherapy, the SANAD trial, showed similar efficacy of carbamazepine, lamotrigine, and oxcarbazepine, but a lower comparative efficacy of gabapentin and topiramate, for treating new-onset focal seizures.[30] In another unblinded randomized study, levetiracetam monotherapy was as effective as controlled-release carbamazepine for focal seizures or extended-release valproic acid/valproate for generalized seizures in patients with new-onset epilepsy.[31]

Tolerability and safety in new-onset epilepsy

Given the similar efficacy of many first-line AEDs in new-onset epilepsy, the comparative tolerability and safety become important rationales in the final choice of an AED. **Table 3** provides an overview of the main tolerability and safety considerations for currently available AEDs.

The evidence base for the comparative tolerability of individual AEDs given as monotherapy is primarily limited to regulatory randomized controlled trials, which typically show a similar proportion of patients with side effects when comparing newer AEDs such as levetiracetam and zonisamide to carbamazepine.[18,32] In addition, regulatory trials are powered for efficacy assessment but are often underpowered to determine differences in tolerability and safety. In the SANAD trial, approximately 50% of patients reported at least one side effect from carbamazepine or valproic acid/valproate as well as from newer AEDs, such as lamotrigine, gabapentin, oxcarbazepine, and topiramate.[33,34] Despite expectations that it may be otherwise, there is thus no compelling evidence that these recently approved AEDs are generally better tolerated than the older AEDs carbamazepine and valproic acid/valproate. With regard to safety, valproic acid/valproate appears to be the most teratogenic AED currently on the market, as pointed out by a recent official ILAE report,[35,36] and valproate is generally seen as a drug of last resort for women who cannot be adequately treated otherwise.[37] Newer AEDs such as gabapentin or levetiracetam cause fewer or no dermatologic hypersensitivity reactions and do not cause the drug interactions seen with older AEDs that can substantially lower the efficacy of other medications, including other AEDs, when taken in combination (see later discussion). In addition, patients may be self-treating with over-the-counter dietary supplements or herbal preparations, some of which may interact with AEDs, such as when gingko biloba or St. John's wort are taken with hepatically metabolized AEDs.[11]

Changing Antiepileptic Drugs Because of Poor Efficacy

For patients who continue to have seizures despite taking the first AED, the physician has 2 options: an alternative monotherapy (substitution) or a combination therapy (add-on), which generally involves adding a second drug to the current monotherapy.[10] Randomized trials,[38,39] albeit small, have not provided evidence of which strategy should be preferred, and both options are used in clinical practice.[40] Although substitution is clearly preferable for patients with serious idiosyncratic side effects from the first AED, many physicians prefer add-on treatment with small dose increments mainly because it avoids the possibility of breakthrough seizures after discontinuation of the baseline drug.[10] In addition, add-on treatment has become easier with modern, nonenzyme-inducing AEDs. It should be noted, however, that currently there are no predictors or biomarkers that the patient will benefit in terms of treatment effect better from a combination treatment or from switching AEDs. Furthermore, and this is astounding, there currently is no evidence that one adjunctive AED is better than another in terms of efficacy. Unfortunately, AED therapy of seizures is still in the era of trial and error. Critics have, somewhat hyperbolically, suggested that a toss of a coin would be just as good to determine which among 2 AEDs will be most efficacious.

Any patient in whom at least 2 trials of adequately dosed AEDs have not brought sustained remission meets the official ILAE criteria for drug-resistant epilepsy.[41] However, this official definition does not specify the number of failed prior lifetime AEDs, which is one of the best predictors of drug resistance,[2,3] and many other clinical definitions exist for different purposes. For example, an influential study considered epilepsy to be drug resistant if treatment for 12 months does not achieve seizure freedom, for whatever reason.[42] With this definition, it has been shown that as many as 36% of newly treated patients have drug-resistant seizures.[42] If the definition of frequent and severe seizures despite optimal treatment is used so that alternative therapies including surgery might be included, only 5% to 10% of newly diagnosed patients are estimated have drug-resistant seizures.[43] Absolute drug resistance may require failure of at least 6 AEDs, as a significant minority of patients (17%) becomes seizure-free by addition of newly administered AEDs even after previous failure of 2 to 5 AEDs to control seizures.[27,44,45] Whatever the best definition may be, these data suggest there is no room for complacency among physicians treating patients who have had persistent seizures over many years. The mechanisms underlying drug-resistant epilepsy still remain to be fully elucidated and are beyond the scope of this article (see Ref.[19]).

For patients whose clinical course meets the minimum ILAE definition of drug-resistant epilepsy,[41] relatively short-term studies show that the chance of seizure freedom declines with successive drug regimens, most markedly from the first to the third AED, especially in patients with localization-related epilepsies.[27] In one representative study from an epilepsy clinic, seizure-free rates decreased from 62% for the first AED to 42% after one prior AED proved ineffective.[44] Among patients who had no response to the first AED, the percentage who subsequently became seizure-free was considerably smaller (11%) when treatment failure was due to lack of efficacy than when it was due to intolerable side effects (41%) or an idiosyncratic reaction (55%).[42] Encouragingly, a longitudinal study encompassing almost 40 years of follow-up found that nearly 4 of 5 patients whose seizures were not initially controlled after 2 trials of suitable AEDs eventually entered one or more 1-year remissions, and half had at least a 5-year remission.[26] Idiopathic or cryptogenic cause was the only significant predictor of entering remission in this study.[26]

Remarkably, there is no class 1 evidence for any of the 25 new AEDs on the market showing superior efficacy for treatment of drug-resistant epilepsy of any definition.[19] In addition, it is disquieting that there is no evidence that modern AEDs have substantially lowered the proportion of patients with drug-resistant epilepsy in recent years.[19] New adjunctive AEDs are only moderately more effective than placebo. (If the AED is not more effective than placebo, the drug gets no marketing access.) In a recent meta-analysis of 54 randomized controlled add-on trials in 11,106 patients with refractory epilepsy, the benefit in efficacy between adding a new AED and adding placebo was only 6% for seizure freedom and 21% for 50% reduction in seizure frequency,[46] suggesting that better strategies for finding more effective antiseizure drugs are needed for refractory epilepsy.

Changing Antiepileptic Drugs Because of Poor Tolerability

Iatrogenic overtreatment (defined as unnecessary drug load) is a leading cause of poor tolerability of AEDs, either by unnecessarily exceeding the recommended dosage for a particular AED or through drug interactions after adding another unnecessary AED.[47] Actual side effects and the patient's perceived risk of side effects or safety risks may compromise adherence to the prescribed dosing schedule. Poor adherence, in turn, may lower AED efficacy, with potentially fatal results[48] and also paradoxically cause heightened or prolonged side effects by not allowing tolerance to side effects to develop.[49]

Therapeutic monitoring

Although target plasma AED concentrations are available for several drugs (**Table 4**), they are clearly less valuable for optimizing AED dosages and dosing schedules than monitoring the patient's clinical course.[10] Except for phenytoin, for which monitoring is strongly recommended, particularly at concentrations greater than 20 mg/L because of the nonlinear saturation dose kinetics, monitoring of other AED plasma concentrations should therefore be individualized to confirm suspected nonadherence or to evaluate unexplained toxicity or uncontrolled seizures.[10] Even so, although therapeutic drug monitoring may improve the benefit-to-risk ratio of AED therapy in some patients, there are many practical limitations.[55] For example, further work is needed to clarify its role in improving seizure control during pregnancy and identifying serum drug concentrations that may be considered safe for fetal exposure.[56] Pharmacogenomics may be helpful in selecting specific AEDs.[57] People of Asian descent carrying the HLA-B*15:02 allele are at significant risk for developing Stevens-Johnson syndrome (SJS)/toxic epidermal necrolysis (TEN) from carbamazepine, lamotrigine, and phenytoin.[58] Screening is thus recommended before starting these AEDs in Han Chinese and Southeast Asians.[59] Drug interaction may cause a drop or an increase in serum concentration (**Table 5**). If a neurologist prescribes an AED that may affect the serum concentrations of the baseline medication, it is advisable, also from a liability standpoint, to inform the referring physician about the change in medication.

The Elderly

The age-related change in pharmacokinetics and higher sensitivity of the elderly to adverse events of many AEDs associated with aging usually requires more cautious AED selection and dosing in the elderly. Lower glomerular filtration rates should prompt reduced doses of AEDs excreted through the kidneys; body fat, albumin, and cytochrome p450 changes also occur, and oxcarbazepine-related hyponatremia may be more frequent.[10,60] In addition, concomitant diseases, such as hypertension, are frequent and often require medications, including diuretics, increasing the possibility of hyponatremia, and drug interactions with AEDs. AED monotherapy and the use of well-tolerated AEDs that are not associated with drug interactions, such as gabapentin and lamotrigine,[61] low-dose topiramate,[62] and levetiracetam (no evidence class I study available), are preferable. In addition, adherence to AED regimens may be more difficult in the elderly with cognitive decline.

Stopping Antiepileptic Drug Treatment

Patients who become seizure-free on therapy and remain so for a prolonged period may understandably wish to discontinue treatment. The decision to discontinue AEDs should be based on the individual's risk of seizure recurrence after discontinuing AEDs, which, overall, is 2-fold higher for the following 2 years off of AEDs compared with staying on drugs and returns to the relapse risk of those staying on AEDs (**Table 6**).

Table 4
Dosages and effective plasma concentrations of antiepileptic drugs for the treatment of epilepsy in adults

AED	Suggested Titration	Suggested Range of Average Target Dose (Total mg/d; Frequency of Dosing)	Target Plasma Concentration (mg/L)
Carbamazepine	200 mg every 3 d	600–1200 bid or tid	3–12
Clobazam	10 mg per day	10–60 mg BID or qd	Na
Eslicarbazepine	400 mg every 3–7 d	800–1200	Na
Felbamate	300 mg every 7 d	2400–3600 bid, tid	20–45
Gabapentin	300 mg every 1–3 d	900–3600 bid, tid	Na
Lacosamide	100 mg every 3–7 d	400–600 bid	Na
Lamotrigine	Monotherapy: 25 mg for 2 wk, 50 mg for the next 2 wk, then increases of 50–100 mg/wk. Add-on in the presence of valproate: 25 mg every other day for 2 wk, 25 mg/d for the next 2 wk, then increases of 25–50 mg/wk. Add-on in the presence of enzyme-inducing AEDs: 50 mg for 2 wk, 100 mg for the next 2 wk, then increases of 50–100 mg/wk	100–400 qd, bid	2–15
Levetiracetam	500 mg every 1–3 d	1000–3000 bid	Na
Oxcarbazepine	150 mg every 3–7 d	800–1800 bid, tid	7.5–20 (MHD)
Phenobarbital	50 mg every 7 d	50–200 qd, bid	10–40
Phenytoin	50–100 mg every 3–5 d; beyond 200 mg in 25–30 mg steps	200–300 bid, tid, qd for extended release availability	5–25
Perampanel	2 mg every 3–7 d	8–12 qd	Na
Pregabalin	75–150 mg every 3–7 d	150–600 bid, tid	Na
Primidone	62.5–250 mg every 7 d	500–750 bid, tid	10–40 (PHB)
Retigabine	100 mg/d increased by 150 mg/d	900–1200 bid, tid	Na
Tiagabine	6 mg every 5–7 d	36–60 bid, tid	Na
Topiramate	25 mg for 1–2 wk; beyond 100 mg, 25–50 mg per week	100–400 bid, tid	Na
Vigabatrin	500 mg every 7 d	500–3000 bid	Na
Valproate	500 mg every 3–7 d	600–1500 bid slow release	40–120
Zonisamide	100 mg ever 3–7 d	200–600 bid, tid	Na

Abbreviations: bid, 2 times per day; MHD, monohydroxy metabolite; Na, irrelevant; PHB, phenobarbital; qd, once a day; tid, 3 times per day.

Adapted from Schmidt D, Schachter SC. Drug treatment of epilepsy in adults. BMJ 2014;348:g2546; and *Modified from* Schmidt D. Drug treatment of epilepsy: options and limitations. Epilepsy Behav 2009;15:56–65; and Faught E. Ezogabine: a new angle on potassium gates. Epilepsy Curr 2011;11:75–8.

Table 5
Simplified synopsis of drug interaction properties of common antiepileptic drugs

AED	Clinically Relevant Interactions When Added to Other Drugs Including AEDs	Clinically Relevant Interactions When Other Drugs Are Added
Clobazam (CLB)	No relevant change	No relevant change
Felbamate (FBM)	Increases plasma concentrations of VPA, PHT, PB, CBZ epoxide	Plasma concentration reduced by enzyme inducers
Gabapentin (GBP)	No relevant change	No relevant change
Levetiracetam (LEV)	No relevant change	No relevant change
Lacosamide (LCM)	No relevant change	Plasma concentration reduced by enzyme inducers
Zonisamide (ZNS)	No relevant change	Plasma concentration reduced by enzyme inducers
Topiramate (TPM)	No relevant change	Plasma concentration reduced by enzyme inducers
Carbamazepine (CBZ)	Lower plasma concentrations of LTG, TGB, VPA and lower efficacy of other drugs[a]	Plasma concentration increased by a variety of drugs, including erythromycin, propoxyphene, isoniazid, cimetidine, verapamil, diltiazem, fluoxetine
Eslicarbazepine (ESL)	Lower plasma concentrations and lower efficacy of other drugs[a]	Plasma concentration reduced by enzyme inducers
Ethosuximide (ETS)	Uncertain	Plasma concentration reduced by enzyme inducers
Lamotrigine (LTG)	No relevant change	Plasma concentration increased by valproate and reduced by enzyme inducers
Oxcarbazepine (OXC)	Lower plasma concentrations of LTG, PHT, TGB, VPA and lower efficacy of other drugs[a] at OXC doses of >900 mg[a]	Plasma concentration reduced by enzyme inducers
Perampanel (PER)	No relevant change	Plasma concentration reduced by enzyme inducers
Phenobarbital (PHB)	Lower plasma concentrations of LTG, OXC, PHT, TGB, VPA and lower efficacy of other drugs[a]	Plasma concentration increased by valproate and felbamate
Phenytoin (PHT)[a]	Lower plasma concentrations of LTG, PHT, TGB, VPA and lower efficacy of other drugs[a]	VPA competes for protein binding
Pregabalin	No relevant change	No relevant change
Primidone (PRM)	Lower plasma concentrations of LTG, OXC, PHT, TGB, VPA, and others. Lower efficacy of other drugs[a]	Plasma concentration reduced by enzyme inducers
Retigabine (RTG)	No relevant change	No relevant change
Valproate (VPA)	Higher toxicity of PHT, PHB, and PRM[b]	Plasma concentration reduced by enzyme inducers
Vigabatrin (VGB)	No relevant change	No relevant change

[a] Inducers of cytochrome P 450 enzyme system.
[b] Inhibitor of Uridin-diphosphate-Glucuronyl-Transferase System and the need to monitor serum concentrations. Italics indicate non-enzymeinducing agents.
Data from Refs.[10,23,50–54]

Table 6	
Stopping antiepileptic drugs in patients in remission	
High-Risk Profile for Seizure Recurrence Off AEDs[63]	**When May It Be Safe to Discontinue?[64]**

• Being 16 y or older
• Taking more than one AED
• Having seizures after starting AED therapy
• History of generalized tonic–clonic seizures
• History of myoclonic seizures
• Having an abnormal EEG in prior year
	• Seizure freedom >2 y implies 60% chance of persistent remission in certain epilepsy syndromes
	• Favorable factors:
	  ○ Control easily achieved on a low dose of one drug
	  ○ No previous unsuccessful attempts at withdrawal
	  ○ Normal neurologic examination and EEG
	  ○ Primary generalized epilepsy except juvenile myoclonic epilepsy
	  ○ Benign syndromes

Considerations include driving, pregnancy, work, and family.

Adapted from Medical Research Council Antiepileptic Drug Withdrawal Study Group. Prognostic index for recurrence of seizures after remission of epilepsy. BMJ 1993;306:1376; and American Academy of Neurology Practice parameter: a guideline for discontinuing antiepileptic drugs in seizure-free patients—summary statement. Neurology 1996;47:602.

Other studies suggest the risk of seizure recurrence off of AEDs may be as high as 34% (95% confidence interval: 27–43), with a wide range of 12% to 66%,[65] and perhaps somewhat higher in adults (39%) than in children (31%).[66] Other considerations are that a recurrent seizure once AEDs are stopped may be embarrassing and stigmatizing for many patients and has the potential for loss of driver's license or, rarely, even accidental or seizure-related death. Furthermore, it is disconcerting that restarting AEDs after a seizure recurrence does not guarantee immediate and sustained remission.[39,67] On the other hand, the impact of ongoing AED-related side effects and drug interactions may argue in favor of AED discontinuation. It may thus be advisable to cautiously offer discontinuation using a slow taper schedule in suitable patients after a thorough and documented discussion of the pros and cons. Although outside of the scope of this article, this recommendation also applies to stopping AEDs for patients in seizure remission following epilepsy surgery.[68,69]

SUMMARY AND LOOKING AHEAD

Most patients with epilepsy will achieve lasting remission of seizures on generally well-tolerated antiseizure drug therapy. The introduction of many new AEDs over the last 2 to 3 decades has brought more treatment options. Nevertheless, approximately 20% of patients continue to suffer from uncontrolled seizures despite all available pharmacologic options, and even more are at significant risk of neuropsychiatric comorbidities. New medications are urgently needed with fewer side effects and better efficacy compared with available AEDs. In addition, there is a need for antiepileptogenic and disease-modifying agents. Because many large pharmaceutical companies have stopped innovating in this therapeutic area, it is becoming increasingly important for foundations and government agencies to fund discovery of new AEDs, and to do so at a level commensurate with the prevalence and costs of drug-resistant epilepsy. Novel approaches to the development of new drugs are emerging[23] that offer hope toward finding more effective antiseizure drugs to treat ongoing drug-resistant epilepsy, antiepileptogenic agents to prevent symptomatic or genetic epilepsy before the first seizure, and disease-modifying agents to mitigate established epilepsy.[23]

REFERENCES

1. Berg AT, Berkovic SF, Brodie MJ, et al. Revised terminology and concepts for organization of seizures and epilepsies: report of the ILAE Commission on Classification and Terminology, 2005–2009. Epilepsia 2010;51:676–85.
2. Cockerell OC, Johnson AL, Sander JW, et al. Prognosis of epilepsy: a review and further analysis of the first nine years of the British National General Practice Study of Epilepsy, a prospective population-based study. Epilepsia 1997;38(1):31–46.
3. Sillanpää M, Schmidt D. Natural history of treated childhood-onset epilepsy: prospective, long-term population-based study. Brain 2006;129(Pt 3):617–24.
4. Sillanpää M, Schmidt D. Epilepsy: long-term rates of childhood-onset epilepsy remission confirmed. Nat Rev Neurol 2015;11(3):130–1.
5. Kim LG, Johnson TL, Marson AG, et al, MRC MESS Study Group. Prediction of risk of seizure recurrence after a single seizure and early epilepsy: further results from the MESS trial. Lancet Neurol 2006;5:317–22.
6. Schmidt D. AED development in treatment of epilepsy. In: Shorvon S, Perucca E, Engel J, editors. Chapter 4. New York: Wiley; 2015. p. 61–74.
7. Fisher RS, Acevedo C, Arzimanoglou A, et al. ILAE official report: a practical clinical definition of epilepsy. Epilepsia 2014;55(4):475–82.
8. Hauser WA, Rich SS, Lee JR, et al. Risk of recurrent seizures after two unprovoked seizures. N Engl J Med 1998;338:429–34.
9. Marson AG. When to start antiepileptic drug treatment and with what evidence? Epilepsia 2008;49(Suppl 9):3–6.
10. Schmidt D. Drug treatment of epilepsy: options and limitations. Epilepsy Behav 2009;15:56–65.
11. Schmidt D, Schachter SC. Drug treatment of epilepsy in adults. BMJ 2014;348: g2546.
12. Mattson RH, Cramer JA, Collins JF, et al. Comparison of carbamazepine, phenobarbital, phenytoin, and primidone in partial and secondarily generalized tonic-clonic seizures. N Engl J Med 1985;313:145–51.
13. Glauser TA, Cnaan A, Shinnar S, et al. Childhood Absence Epilepsy Study Group. Ethosuximide, valproic acid, and lamotrigine in childhood absence epilepsy. N Engl J Med 2010;362(9):790–9.
14. Kwan P, Brodie MJ. Early identification of refractory epilepsy. N Engl J Med 2000; 342:314–9.
15. Glauser T, Ben-Menachem E, Bourgeois B, et al. Updated ILAE evidence review of antiepileptic drug efficacy and effectiveness as initial monotherapy for epileptic seizures and syndromes. Epilepsia 2013;54(3):551–63.
16. Chadwick D. Safety and efficacy of vigabatrin and carbamazepine in newly diagnosed epilepsy: a multicentre randomised double-blind study. Vigabatrin European Monotherapy Study Group. Lancet 1999;354(9172):13–9.
17. Chadwick DW (1), Anhut H, Greiner MJ, et al. A double-blind trial of gabapentin monotherapy for newly diagnosed partial seizures. International Gabapentin Monotherapy Study Group 945-77. Neurology 1998;51(5):1282–8.
18. Baulac M, Brodie MJ, Patten A, et al. Efficacy and tolerability of zonisamide versus controlled-release carbamazepine for newly diagnosed partial epilepsy: a phase 3, randomised, double-blind, non-inferiority trial. Lancet Neurol 2012;11(7):579–88.

19. Löscher W, Schmidt D. Modern antiepileptic drug development has failed to deliver: ways out of the current dilemma. Epilepsia 2011;52:657–78.
20. Rogawski MA, Löscher W. The neurobiology of antiepileptic drugs. Nat Rev Neurosci 2004;5:553–64.
21. Bialer M, White HS. Key factors in the discovery and development of new antiepileptic drugs. Nat Rev Drug Discov 2010;9:68–82.
22. Abou-Khalil B, Schmidt D. Antiepileptic drugs: advantages and disadvantages. In: Stefan H, Theodore WH, editors. Handbook of clinical neurology, vol. 108. Epilepsy part II: treatment. Amsterdam: Elsevier; 2012. p. 723–39.
23. Löscher W, Klitgaard H, Twyman RE, et al. New avenues for anti-epileptic drug discovery and development. Nat Rev Drug Discov 2013;12(10):757–76.
24. Prosser H, Almond S, Walley T. Influences on GPs' decision to prescribe new drugs—the importance of who says what. Fam Pract 2003;20(1):61–8.
25. Greiner W, Witte J. AMNOG-Report 2015—Nutzenbewertung von Arzneimitteln in Deutschland. Heidelberg (Germany): medhochzwei Verlag; 2015.
26. Sillanpää M, Schmidt D. Early seizure frequency and aetiology predict long-term medical outcome in childhood-onset epilepsy. Brain 2009;132:989–98.
27. Brodie MJ, Barry SJ, Bamagous GA, et al. Patterns of treatment response in newly diagnosed epilepsy. Neurology 2012;78:1548–54.
28. Proposal for revised clinical and electroencephalographic classification of epileptic seizures. Commission on classification and terminology of the International League Against Epilepsy. Epilepsia 1981;22(4):489–501.
29. Costa J, Fareleira F, Ascencao R, et al. Clinical comparability of the new antiepileptic drugs in refractory partial epilepsy: a systematic review and meta-analysis. Epilepsia 2011;52(7):1280–91.
30. Bonnett L, Smith CT, Smith D, et al. Prognostic factors for time to treatment failure and time to 12 months of remission for patients with focal epilepsy: posthoc, subgroup analyses of data from the SANAD trial. Lancet Neurol 2012; 11(4):331–40.
31. Trinka E, Marson AG, Van Paesschen W, et al. KOMET: an unblinded, randomised, two parallel-group, stratified trial comparing the effectiveness of levetiracetam with controlled-release carbamazepine and extended-release sodium valproate as monotherapy in patients with newly diagnosed epilepsy. J Neurol Neurosurg Psychiatry 2013;84:1138–47.
32. Brodie MJ, Perucca E, Ryvlin P, et al, Levetiracetam Monotherapy Study Group. Comparison of levetiracetam and controlled-release carbamazepine in newly diagnosed epilepsy. Neurology 2007;68(6):402–8.
33. Marson AG, Al-Kharusi AM, Alwaidh M, et al. The SANAD study of effectiveness of valproate, lamotrigine, or topiramate for generalised and unclassifiable epilepsy: an unblinded randomised controlled trial. Lancet 2007;369:1016–26.
34. Marson AG, Al-Kharusi AM, Alwaidh M, et al. The SANAD study of effectiveness of carbamazepine, gabapentin, lamotrigine, oxcarbazepine, or topiramate for treatment of partial epilepsy: an unblinded randomised controlled trial. Lancet 2007;369:1000–15.
35. Tomson T, Marson A, Boon P, et al. Valproate in the treatment of epilepsy in girls and women of childbearing potential. Epilepsia 2015;56(7):1006–19.
36. Meador KJ, Baker GA, Browning N, et al. Fetal antiepileptic drug exposure and cognitive outcomes at age 6 years (NEAD study): a prospective observational study. Lancet Neurol 2013;12(3):244–52.
37. Schmidt D. The dilemma of treating young women with generalized epilepsy with sodium valproate and how to get out of it. Seizure 2015;24:143–4.

38. Deckers CLP, Hekster YA, Keyser A, et al. Monotherapy versus polytherapy for epilepsy: a multicenter double-blind randomized study. Epilepsia 2001;42: 1387–94.
39. Beghi E, Gatti G, Tonini C, et al. Adjunctive therapy versus alternative monotherapy in patients with partial epilepsy failing on a single drug: a multicentre, randomized, pragmatic controlled trial. Epilepsy Res 2003;57:1–13.
40. Karceski S, Morrell MJ, Carpenter D. Treatment of epilepsy in adults: expert opinion, 2005. Epilepsy Behav 2005;7:S1–64.
41. Kwan P, Arzimanoglou A, Berg AT, et al. Definition of drug resistant epilepsy: consensus proposal by the ad hoc task force of the ILAE Commission on Therapeutic Strategies. Epilepsia 2010;51(6):1069–77.
42. Kwan P, Brodie MJ. Early identification of refractory epilepsy. N Engl J Med 2000; 342(5):314–9.
43. Hauser WA. The natural history of drug resistant epilepsy: epidemiologic considerations. Epilepsy Res Suppl 1992;5:25–8.
44. Schiller Y, Najjar Y. Quantifying the response to antiepileptic drugs: effect of past treatment history. Neurology 2008;70:54–65.
45. Sillanpää M, Schmidt D. Is incident drug-resistance of childhood-onset epilepsy reversible? A long-term follow-up study. Brain 2012;135(Pt 7):2256–62.
46. Beyenburg S, Stavem K, Schmidt D. Placebo-corrected efficacy of modern antiepileptic drugs for refractory epilepsy: systematic review and meta-analysis. Epilepsia 2010;51:7–26.
47. Schmidt D. Strategies to prevent overtreatment with antiepileptic drugs in patients with epilepsy. Epilepsy Res 2002;52(1):61–9.
48. Faught E, Duh MS, Weiner JR, et al. Nonadherence to antiepileptic drugs and increased mortality: findings from the RANSOM Study. Neurology 2008;71(20): 1572–8.
49. Löscher W, Schmidt D. Experimental and clinical evidence for loss of effect (tolerance) during prolonged treatment with antiepileptic drugs. Epilepsia 2006;47: 1253–84.
50. Faught E. Ezogabine: a new angle on potassium gates. Epilepsy Curr 2011;11: 75–8.
51. Benedetti MS. Enzyme induction and inhibition by new antiepileptic drugs: a review of human studies. Fundam Clin Pharmacol 2000;14:301–19.
52. Patsalos PN, Perucca E. Clinically important drug interactions in epilepsy: general features and interactions between antiepileptic drugs. Lancet Neurol 2003; 2:347–56.
53. Strolin-Benedetti M. Enzyme induction and inhibition by new antiepileptic drugs: a review of human studies. Fundam Clin Pharmacol 2000;14:301–9.
54. Kousar S, Wafai ZA, Wani MA, et al. Clinical relevance of genetic polymorphism in CYP2C9 gene to pharmacodynamics and pharmacokinetics of phenytoin in epileptic patients: validatory pharmacogenomic approach to pharmacovigilance. Int J Clin Pharmacol Ther 2015;53(7):504–16.
55. Patsalos PN, Berry DJ, Bourgeois BF, et al. Antiepileptic drugs–best practice guidelines for therapeutic drug monitoring: a position paper by the subcommission on therapeutic drug monitoring, ILAE Commission on Therapeutic Strategies. Epilepsia 2008;49(7):1239–76.
56. Adab N. Therapeutic monitoring of antiepileptic drugs during pregnancy and in the postpartum period: is it useful? CNS Drugs 2006;20(10):791–800.
57. Löscher W, Klotz U, Zimprich F, et al. The clinical impact of pharmacogenetics on the treatment of epilepsy. Epilepsia 2009;50(1):1–23.

58. Illing PT, Vivian JP, Purcell AW, et al. Human leukocyte antigen-associated drug hypersensitivity. Curr Opin Immunol 2013;25(1):81–9.
59. Cheung YK, Cheng SH, Chan EJ, et al. HLA-B alleles associated with severe cutaneous reactions to antiepileptic drugs in Han Chinese. Epilepsia 2013; 54(7):1307–14.
60. Robertson MM, Trimble MR. The treatment of depression in patients with epilepsy. A double-blind trial. J Affect Disord 1985;9(2):127–36.
61. Rowan AJ, Ramsay RE, Collins JF, et al. New onset geriatric epilepsy: a randomized study of gabapentin, lamotrigine, and carbamazepine. Neurology 2005;64: 1868–73.
62. Ramsay RE, Uthman B, Pryor FM, et al. Topiramate in older patients with partial-onset seizures: a pilot double-blind, dose-comparison study. Epilepsia 2008;49: 1180–5.
63. Prognostic index for recurrence of seizures after remission of epilepsy. Medical research council antiepileptic drug withdrawal study group. BMJ 1993;306:1374–8.
64. Practice parameter: a guideline for discontinuing antiepileptic drugs in seizure-free patients—summary statement. Report of the quality standards subcommittee of the American Academy of Neurology. Neurology 1996;47:600–2.
65. Schmidt D, Löscher W. Uncontrolled epilepsy following discontinuation of antiepileptic drugs in seizure-free patients: a review of current clinical experience. Acta Neurol Scand 2005;111(5):291–300.
66. Berg AT, Shinnar S. Relapse following discontinuation of antiepileptic drugs: a meta-analysis. Neurology 1994;44(4):601–8.
67. Bonnett LJ, Shukralla A, Tudur-Smith C, et al. Seizure recurrence after antiepileptic drug withdrawal and the implications for driving: further results from the MRC Antiepileptic Drug Withdrawal Study and a systematic review. J Neurol Neurosurg Psychiatry 2011;82(12):1328–33.
68. Schmidt D, Baumgartner C, Löscher W. Seizure recurrence after planned discontinuation of antiepileptic drugs in seizure-free patients after epilepsy surgery: a review of current clinical experience. Epilepsia 2004;45(2):179–86.
69. Braun KPJ, Schmidt D. Stopping antiepileptic drugs in seizure-free patients. Curr Opin Neurol 2014;27(2):219–26.

Methods for Measuring Seizure Frequency and Severity

Anahita Aghaei-Lasboo, MD, Robert S. Fisher, MD, PhD*

KEYWORDS

- Seizures • Epilepsy • Diaries • Seizure severity • Seizure detection

KEY POINTS

- The clinical practice of epilepsy is based in significant part on counting seizures and assessing their severity, but methods for accomplishing these tasks are limited.
- Seizure severity scales are subjective and may not account for individual tolerance of consequences of seizures.
- People may be unaware of their seizures, so many seizures go unreported. Even if noted, seizures may not be logged accurately in a diary.
- Video-electroencephalogram (EEG) monitoring is accurate but time-limited, done in an artificial setting, and expensive. Seizures seen on EEG may or may not have a clinical correlate.
- Biosensors, such as accelerometers to detect shaking or electrodermal response (EDR), can be useful but have limited sensitivity and specificity. Better methods are needed.

INTRODUCTION

The clinical practice of epilepsy is based in significant part on counting and tracking seizures, even though the spectrum of epilepsy extends far beyond seizures.[1] Seizure characteristics of potential interest include seizure frequency, duration, severity, time of day, and response to precipitating factors. Unfortunately, recent studies indicate that the quality of information as reported by some patients and caregivers is low.[2,3] This article reviews possible approaches to tracking seizure frequency and severity. None of them is ideal in all circumstances, and therefore a variety of available approaches should be used. **Box 1** lists some common and potential near-future methods for tracking seizure occurrence or severity.

Disclosures: R.S. Fisher holds stock in Advanced Neurometrics, Inc., Avails Medical, ICVRx and Zeto, Inc., and is supported by the James and Carrie Anderson fund for Epilepsy Research, The Maslah Saul MD Chair, the Steve Chen Epilepsy fund, and the Susan Horngren fund.
Stanford Neuroscience Health Center, 213 Quarry Road, Room 2852, Palo Alto, CA 94304-5979, USA
* Corresponding author.
E-mail address: robert.fisher@stanford.edu

Neurol Clin 34 (2016) 383–394
http://dx.doi.org/10.1016/j.ncl.2015.11.001
0733-8619/16/$ – see front matter © 2016 Elsevier Inc. All rights reserved.

neurologic.theclinics.com

Box 1
Methods for tracking seizures

Severity scales
  Liverpool Seizure Severity Scale, and PIES)
  National Hospital Seizure Severity Scale (Chalfont)
  Personal Impact of Epilepsy Scale (PIES)

Seizure diaries

Shake detectors
  Wrist accelerometers
  Bed shake monitor
  Strap or belt shake detector
  Smartphone accelerometers
  Surface EMG

Electrodermal response (EDR)

EEG monitoring
  Ambulatory EEG
  Inpatient video-EEG
  Dry EEG
  Recordings from implanted devices

SEIZURE SEVERITY SCALES

Seizure severity can be assessed along several dimensions, some subjective and others objective. There is no universally applicable scale, because an individual who is well accustomed to generalized tonic-clonic seizures (GTCSs) might consider those seizures less severe than would an individual with infrequent but disabling focal seizures.[4] The traditional method for measuring seizure severity involves completion of several validated questionnaires or reporting devices. Some of these are completed by an individual with epilepsy or by a family and others by medical personnel in an interview mode.

The Liverpool Seizure Severity Scale[5,6] was designed to measure patients' perceptions of changes in their seizure severity. The original scale comprised 16 items, with 6 items assaying perception of control over the seizures (including ability to predict seizures, ability to fight off the seizures, having an aura, having control over the seizures, and prevention of normal activities), and 10 items pertaining to the ictal or the postictal severity (including overall subjective severity, loss of consciousness, severity and duration of postictal confusion, falls associated with seizures, postictal sleepiness, postictal headache, incontinence, tongue biting, and other injuries). Each item was scored on a 1-point to 4-point scale. Reliability and validity were documented during clinical drug trials and in other settings. The original Liverpool Seizure Severity Scale was limited in its comprehensiveness, responsiveness, and application in patients with multiple types of seizures. To make the scale more comprehensive, an additional 4 items were later added to the percept subscale (timing during the day, seizures in sleep only, and seizure clustering vs random seizures) and to the ictal/postictal subscale (lip smacking and fidgeting). The responsiveness of the scale was enhanced by increasing the evaluation range from 0 to 4 and providing a 5-item response choice instead of 4 for 4 of the subscale items: presence of aura, duration of postictal confusion, loss of consciousness, and time to full recovery. The goal was to make the items more sensitive to differentiating between simple partial seizures and complex partial seizures (CPSs). The patients were also asked to complete the scale for the least and most severe types of their seizures.[7]

The Chalfont Seizure Severity Scale,[4] later renamed the National Hospital Seizure Severity Scale,[8] is a patient-based and observer scale that was developed to measure severity of the seizures, for different types of seizures, based on the most subjectively disturbing aspects of the seizure. The scale is completed by those who observe the seizure and is also based on responses obtained from the patient. Scoring is performed for "loss of awareness" versus "warning," dropping/spilling a held object, falling to the ground, having an injury, incontinence, automatism, convulsion for duration of the seizure, and time to return to normal. If the seizures occur in sleep, the total score is divided by 2.

In 1983, Cramer and colleagues[9] developed a seizure severity scale for use in the landmark Veterans Administration Cooperative Study Group antiepileptic drug trial.[10] In decreasing order of prevalence, The questionnaire surveyed disturbance in cognitive function; sedation; psychological problems; tremor; drug-related headache; gait problems, abnormal walking; drug-related dizziness/lightheadedness; dysarthria; diplopia; gain or loss of weight; changes in hair; gastrointestinal problems; arthralgia; dental problem; and skin reaction to drug.[11]

A few scales designed to assess global impact of epilepsy incorporate subsections pertaining to seizure severity. A self-assessed patient-oriented outcome scale called the Personal Impact of Epilepsy Scale (PIES)[12] asks 25 questions, 8 of which pertain to some aspect of seizure severity. Bothersome postictal symptoms showed the greatest inverse correlation with quality of life, exceeding even the impact on quality of life produced by seizure-provoked injuries.[13] A seizure severity scale particularly applicable to children with epilepsy is called the Hague Seizure Severity Scale.[14,15]

Seizure severity scales are valid measures but must be interpreted in a clinical context. The greatest severity of some seizures may not relate to the intensity of shaking or its duration or even injuries produced by seizures but by provocation of comorbid factors, such as depression,[16–18] prolonged postictal disability,[19] and limits on daily activities. Capturing the impact of these factors in a concise scale applicable to a diverse population can be challenging.

SEIZURE DIARIES

The traditional method of recording seizures is by subjective documentation in a paper-based calendar diary. Validity of a seizure diary first requires that a patient or family member recognizes occurrence of a seizure, and this is often not the case.[20–22] Even patients with GTCSs may be unaware of having had a recent seizure, because of disrupted memory and postictal confusion. Several studies have documented limited correlation of seizure diaries with other objective methods.[2,23–26]

Adherence with entering seizure reports into a diary can be low. One study[24] evaluated 32 people with drug-resistant partial seizures and found an approximately 50% discrepancy between the people with epilepsy and their caregivers, with fewer seizures reported by caregivers. Test-retest accuracy was studied by Neugebauer,[25] who made phone calls to patients querying the number of seizures on a previous day, comparing phone interview responses to diary entries. Of 84 subjects who reported seizures, 30 of them did not enter the seizure into the diary. Inaccuracy can occur in the other direction, when patients record events they interpret as seizures but are not seizures.

Electronic recording methods might improve accuracy of seizure diaries,[2,23,27,28] and a few studies indicate that they are preferred by some patients.[26] A significant proportion of the population, however, does not have the economic means to own computers or smartwatches nor has experience using them.

Several diaries accessible via the Internet are in current use. The 2 with largest numbers of users are *My Epilepsy Diary* at http://www.epilepsy.com/get-help/my-epilepsy-diary and *Seizure Tracker*, accessible at http://www.seizuretracker.com. At time of this writing, more than 20,000 individuals have used each of these 2 diaries. **Fig. 1** shows a screenshot from one of the diaries. The Epilepsy Foundation has recently introduced My Seizure Diary at http://www.epilepsy.com/get-help/my-epilepsy-diary.

The diaries provide opportunities to enter occurrence of a seizure on a calendar day and describe characteristics of that seizure. Information also can be tracked on side effects of medication, whether medications were missed or taken in extra doses, mood, provoking factors, and other characteristics describing the seizures. Information can be displayed in summary chart form or graphically and communicated with permission to the medical care team. Input into the diaries can be by computer or increasingly by smartphone entry. Such diary information is less likely to be misplaced then a paper diary, and electronic diaries are easier to summarize and analyze. Anonymous population information can be used to describe global characteristics of seizures based on information extracted from online diaries.[28] Electronic diaries, however, exhibit the same drawbacks as do paper diaries regarding lack of awareness of seizures and poor adherence to diary entry.

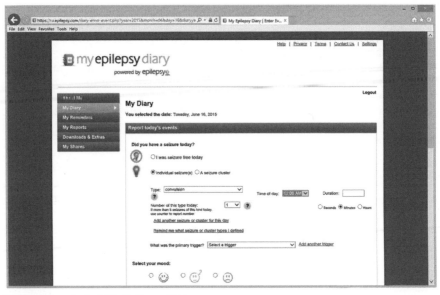

Fig. 1. Screenshot of *My Epilepsy Diary.*

SHAKE DETECTORS

Tonic-clonic seizures are associated with characteristic rhythmic shaking of the extremities in a pattern recognizable to every experienced epilepsy clinician. The initial tonic stiffening entails a relatively high-frequency vibration, which then increases in amplitude and decreases in frequency over time to the clonic phase, followed by cessation of movement. Software can be programmed to register this or other patterns of shaking as detected by accelerometers attached to the patient. Initial experiences with use of accelerometers to detect tonic-clonic seizures was provided by Conradsen and colleagues,[29] Cuppens and colleagues,[30] and Nijsen and colleagues.[31] Characteristic and detectable movement patterns were also produced by some myoclonic, tonic and clonic seizures.[31]

A bed shake monitor by MedPage[32] was able to identify 5 of 8 tonic-clonic seizures but with an unacceptably high false-positive rate of 269 non–seizure-related alarms. Movement can be recorded by straps on the chest or belts, as with the Cyberonics (Houston, TX) ProGuardian system or the RTI Mobile Seizure Alert System (Research Triangle Park, NC).

Accelerometers can be conveniently attached to an arm or leg.[33] Three studies[34–36] documented reasonable sensitivity and specificity of wrist-worn accelerometers. One of these, named SmartWatch (Smart-Monitor.com), is currently commercially available as a shake detector and is undergoing evaluation as a seizure detector. An important feature of wrist shake detectors is availability of a cancel button on a short delay loop. Without this feature, normal activities, such as scratching or brushing teeth, would result in a seizure alarm. The pattern of movement captured by a wristband monitor may be able to distinguish epileptic from nonepileptic seizures[33] in an outpatient environment.

Shake detector wristbands can be linked to seizure diaries in the cloud to produce an automated record of tonic-clonic seizures. In one study,[37] an accelerometer-based wrist device detected 6 of 7 tonic-clonic seizures occurring in an epilepsy monitoring unit and successfully logged the detections to a cloud-based epilepsy diary. In contrast, none of these seizures was logged (as patients were instructed to do) in a bedside paper diary.

In addition to more accurate logging of information, accelerometer-based digital systems can provide additional useful data, such as precise time of day of a seizure, duration, and intensity of shaking. Because many widely available smartphones include accelerometers, applications can be written for devices that people with epilepsy may already possess. One example of an application using smartphones is EpDetect (epdetect.com), which monitors a person's movement while a phone is worn on a belt or in a pocket. When a seizure is detected, it activates an audible alarm and sends a short message service (SMS) to a prespecified phone number. A similar product is Seizario (seizario.com).

Motor seizures are expressed as muscle activity and, therefore, can be detected by EMG. A single-channel surface-mounted EMG patch used in 6 patients detected every tonic-clonic seizure with a median latency of 7.6 seconds and a false-positive rate of 1 event per day.[38] Another study of the same device presented a less favorable false-positive detection rate, ranging from 2 to 8 per hour.[39]

ELECTRODERMAL RESPONSE

Accelerometer watches only detect seizures involving shaking, but the most prevalent problematic seizures in adults are partial seizures, either with no movements or movements that are difficult to distinguish from normal activity.[31] Other strategies are required for detection of nonmotor seizures. One such novel strategy is measurement of the electrodermal response (EDR), formerly called the galvanic skin response.

The EDR, mediated by sympathetic cholinergic fibers,[40] reflects emotional state and autonomic nervous system activity.[41] Measurement of EDR has been used in management of psychiatric problems,[42] stress,[43] electroconvulsive therapy,[44] head trauma,[45] coma,[46] and several other conditions.

Seizures are associated with increased autonomic activity.[47] In 1958, Van Buren[48] showed that EDR activated during temporal lobe seizures, reflected as decreased skin resistance, which is equivalent to increased skin conductance, measured in microsiemens (μS). EDR can be measured at the wrist or ankle by wearable devices.[42,49] In 2010, Poh and colleagues[50] demonstrated a sensor in contact with skin was able to detect a surge in the EDR during seizures. They studied 7 patients, 4 with GTCSs and 3 with CPSs. GTCSs were associated with a change in EDR with magnitude often greater than 20 μS, compared with 0.7 μS for CPSs and nonseizure fluctuations of approximately 2 μS, especially during sleep. Further data were collected on 26 subjects wearing a wristband EDR sensor.[51] Physical exercise and stressful cognitive tasks increased the EDR at the wrist from a typical baseline near 0 to approximately 2 μS. An algorithm was developed that was able to automatically detect 15 of 16 generalized tonic-clonic seizures in 7 patients, with a mean of 0.74 false-positive detections per 24 hours. The sensitivity and specificity of detection of CPSs are still under evaluation. An increase of the EDR in the postictal period correlated with EEG suppression, which may be a risk factor for sudden unexpected death in epilepsy.[52]

ELECTROENCEPHALOGRAM MONITORING

Inpatient video-audio-EEG monitoring is the most accurate way to count seizures because it provides simultaneous behavioral and EEG surveillance.[53] Limitations of inpatient recording are short recording times, an artificial environment, and expense. Medications may be withdrawn while in a monitoring unit to provoke seizures for analysis. Seizure counts in a monitoring unit give little information on outpatient seizure frequency.

Ambulatory EEG (aEEG) has been used in the outpatient setting since 1975.[54] Electrodes are glued to the scalp with long-lasting adhesive and conductive electrode gel. Signals are led to a portable recorder, which typically captures 24 or more hours of 4-channel, 8-channel, 16-channel, or 32-channel EEGs. A paper log is kept of events and times for later analysis by the electroencephalographer. The technology has been reviewed.[55] The most common duration of aEEG is for 24 hours, but recordings can continue for much longer, provided that batteries are replaced and electrode gel refreshed. Stefan and colleagues[56] presented a report of 2 patients, recorded respectively for 137 and 160 hours. The prolonged monitoring, instituted after a period of inpatient monitoring, was useful in quantifying a beneficial response to medication. A large aEEG series was reported from Australia.[57] Of a total 324 studies, lasting up to 5 consecutive days, with daily returns for refreshing the device, 36% showed interictal epileptiform activity and 52% recorded events of interest. Management was altered in response to 22% of the studies.

Prolonged contact with EEG electrode gel and glue can be irritating to skin, so efforts have been made to develop dry and comfortable EEG electrodes.[58–65] These dry electrodes can be coupled with broadcasters able to send EEG signals via Bluetooth or Wi-Fi protocols to remote reading devices. **Table 1** lists examples of wireless EEG systems using dry electrodes. Some of these headset EEGs are currently on the market for gaming or other applications; others are under development or no longer available, but none has yet achieved widespread acceptance as a long-term seizure monitor.

Electrodes can be implanted to record electrographic ictal activity. At time of this writing, no implantable EEG system designed primarily for long-term monitoring is available for commercial use, although several are under development. Two devices intended for therapy, made by NeuroVista and NeuroPace, have the ability to perform long-term seizure counting as a byproduct of their therapeutic purpose.

The NeuroVista product was designed to anticipate and notify of imminent seizures. The technology was successfully validated in dogs[66] and extended to patients.[3] Subdural or epidural electrode arrays are implanted near the seizure focus or foci. These

Table 1
Dry electrode EEG devices

Device/Company/Website	Description
Clinical EEG Systems	
ANI-SI by Advanced Neurometrics. http://advancedneurometrics.com	The ANI-SI™ system, developed by Advanced Neurometrics, INC. (ANI), is a hat-like EEG recording system that can conveniently be put on and removed by the patients. This system has been designed for long-term EEG monitoring.
Ahead 200 by Brainscope. http://www.brainscope.com	A scalp adhesive strip with eight electrodes connected to a computer. In head trauma patients, it can display and quantify deviations of brain function from normal.
DryCap for dense EEG recording by NeuroRex. http://www.neurorex.com/	" NeuroRex Inc. is a small medical company in Houston that is developing dense array dry-electrode cap for multimodal integration of EEG applications in neuroscience and epilepsy."
EPOC & EPOC+ by Emotiv. https://emotiv.com	A 14-channel wireless EEG recording headset. The EPOC+ has accelerometry and other sensors.
Enobio by Neuroelectrics. http://www.neuroelectrics.com	A wearable, wireless EEG recording system with cloth and modular electrodes, available in three versions Enobio 8, Enobio 20 and Enobio 32.
Fourier One by Nielsen. https://twitter.com/cannes_lions/status/478867347957383168	A wearable EEG headset designed for analytics of ongoing cognitive processes.
Mynd by NeuroFocus http://www.fastcompany.com/1741403/thinking-cap-mynd-first-dry-iphone-compatible-portable-brain-scanner	A dry wireless EEG headset with dense array sensors, and capable of wireless transmission and interfacing with a Bluetooth-enabled communications device.
Quick-20 Dry EEG Headset by Cognionics. http://cognionics.com	A portable and wearable EEG recording system with a full 10-20 array. Also cap with 64 channels. Recorded data can be streamed wirelessly via Bluetooth or recorded to memory card
Wearable Sensing by Neurable, Inc. http://www.wearablesensing.com	Has 24 sensors at 10-20 electrode positions
Zeto EEG. http://zeto-inc.com/	A compact, self-use EEG device that improves diagnosis and self-management of epilepsy
Limited Channels	
Brain Stethoscope, Stanford, CA. http://news.stanford.edu/news/2013/september/seizure-music-research-092413.html	An external band of electrodes that converts brain wave signals into musical sounds to enable the listener to detect seizure activity in the brain with minimal training
Ear EEG by Mind Solutions. http://www.prnewswire.com/news-releases/mind-solutions-inc-creates-eegbci-device-that-fits-in-your-ear-273903681.html	Mobile EEG / BCI device worn on the ear, like a common Bluetooth cellular device

(continued on next page)

Table 1 *(continued)*	
Device/Company/Website	**Description**
Versus Headset by Sense Labs. Getversus. com	"Versus provides performance brain training through a brain sensing headset and app. Designed by neuroscientists, . . . Increase impulse control, regulate emotions, stay focused, and sleep better"
iBrain by Neurovigil. http://www. neurovigil.com	A single channel portable EEG recording device that can also be used for at-home sleep monitoring. The device is very small in size and can be attached to an elastic head harness.
Muse EEG monitoring headband by InteraXon. www.choosemuse.com	The device can send real-time information to any blue tooth enabled devices and was primary used for meditation purposes.
NeuroSync by Mind Solutions. https:// mindsolutionscorp.com	Smallest Brain Computer Interface device on the market. Sends EEG via Bluetooth.
Qui Vive by Epitel. http://www.epitelinc.com	A single channel stick-on EEG patch for animals or humans
Wireless EEG Headset by IMEC. http:// www2.imec.be/be_en/research/ wearable-health-monitoring.html	A wearable EEG monitor with a seven sensor headset. The device is able to deliver real-time data to Bluetooth-enabled devices.
Gaming EEG Systems	
NeuroTrail by NeuroPro.http://www. neuropro.ch	A wireless headset for recording of EEG, ECG as well as other biometric data. Recorded data is transmitted wirelessly in real-time using Bluetooth and can be used for clinical or gaming applications.
ThinkGear™ AM and **MindWave**™ by NeuroSky. http://store.neurosky.com	Various biosensor headsets that digitalize EEG signals to power the user-interface of games, applications and investigational medical devices.

electrodes carry the EEG information to a subcutaneously implanted detector, which continually runs a seizure prediction algorithm on the data. When criteria are met, the detector sends a wireless signal to a belt pager that can use color or sound to notify a user of a possible impending seizure. To validate event detection as representing true seizures, the belt pager recorded audio at time of the event, which usually allowed post hoc determination of seizure versus no seizure. Devices were implanted in 15 patients and proved effective in several for signaling a seizure warning. Four of the subjects, however, had complications of the procedure (seroma, infection, site irritation, and device migration), emphasizing the invasive nature of the device.

NeuroPace developed a Food and Drug Administration–approved responsive neurostimulation device (RNS).[67–71] Up to 2 strip or depth wire electrodes with 4 contacts each can be located over 1 or 2 brain regions believed involved in seizure initiation. In a preliminary phase, several seizures are recorded and the detection algorithm tuned to the individual pattern of that patient's seizures. Once tuned, the stimulation component is activated, to attempt stimulation-induced disruption of a seizure. The RNS device proved therapeutically effective in reducing seizure frequency in patients with refractory focal and secondarily generalized seizures.[72] A recent study[73] evaluated seizure detections in 82 patients with bilateral temporal responsive neurostimulators, recorded for a mean 4.7 years. Most patients (82%) in this highly select population were found to have bilateral independent temporal seizure origins. The mean time to make this determination of bilaterality was 41.6 days, with a range of 0 to 376 days. Data from implanted RNS devices can be uploaded via the Internet, providing an effective way to track seizures over long periods of time.

The biggest problem with EEG seizure-detection methods is the possibility of poor correspondence between EEG phenomena and clinical seizures. Electrodes in the wrong place may miss some seizures, even if there is capture of others. Even more problematic are EEG events with no obvious clinical correlate. Some patients with implanted RNS devices register thousands of seizure detections each day but only have a small fraction of this number of perceived seizures. Are these seizures truly subclinical or are they subtle, with manifestations that could be detected in the proper circumstances? The answer to this question is currently unknown.

REFERENCES

1. England MJ, Austin JK, Beck V, et al. Epilepsy across the spectrum: promoting health and understanding. Washington, DC: The Natonal Academies Press; 2012.
2. Fisher RS, Blum DE, DiVentura B, et al. Seizure diaries for clinical research and practice: limitations and future prospects. Epilepsy Behav 2012;24(3):304–10.
3. Cook MJ, O'Brien TJ, Berkovic SF, et al. Prediction of seizure likelihood with a long-term, implanted seizure advisory system in patients with drug-resistant epilepsy: a first-in-man study. Lancet Neurol 2013;12(6):563–71.
4. Duncan JS, Sander JW. The Chalfont Seizure Severity Scale. J Neurol Neurosurg Psychiatr 1991;54(10):873–6.
5. Baker GA, Smith DF, Dewey M, et al. The development of a seizure severity scale as an outcome measure in epilepsy. Epilepsy Res 1991;8(3):245–51.
6. Smith DF, Baker GA, Dewey M, et al. Seizure frequency, patient-perceived seizure severity and the psychosocial consequences of intractable epilepsy. Epilepsy Res 1991;9(3):231–41.
7. Baker GA, Smith DF, Jacoby A, et al. Liverpool seizure severity scale revisited. Seizure 1998;7(3):201–5.
8. O'Donoghue MF, Duncan JS, Sander JW. The National Hospital Seizure Severity Scale: a further development of the Chalfont Seizure Severity Scale. Epilepsia 1996;37(6):563–71.
9. Cramer JA, Smith DB, Mattson RH, et al. A method of quantification for the evaluation of antiepileptic drug therapy. Neurology 1983;33(3 Suppl 1):26–37.
10. Mattson RH, Cramer JA, Collins JF, et al. Comparison of carbamazepine, phenobarbital, phenytoin, and primidone in partial and secondarily generalized tonic-clonic seizures. N Engl J Med 1985;313(3):145–51.
11. Cramer JA, Steinborn B, Striano P, et al. Non-interventional surveillance study of adverse events in patients with epilepsy. Acta Neurol Scand 2011;124(1):13–21.
12. Fisher RS, Nune G, Roberts SE, et al. The personal impact of epilepsy scale (PIES). Epilepsy Behav 2015;42:140–6.
13. Harden CL, Maroof DA, Nikolov B, et al. The effect of seizure severity on quality of life in epilepsy. Epilepsy Behav 2007;11(2):208–11.
14. Carpay HA, Arts WF. Outcome assessment in epilepsy: available rating scales for adults and methodological issues pertaining to the development of scales for childhood epilepsy. Epilepsy Res 1996;24(3):127–36.

15. Carpay HA, Arts WF, Vermeulen J, et al. Parent-completed scales for measuring seizure severity and severity of side-effects of antiepileptic drugs in childhood epilepsy: development and psychometric analysis. Epilepsy Res 1996;24(3): 173–81.
16. Cramer JA, Blum D, Reed M, et al. The influence of comorbid depression on quality of life for people with epilepsy. Epilepsy Behav 2003;4(5):515–21.
17. Cramer JA, Blum D, Reed M, et al. The influence of comorbid depression on seizure severity. Epilepsia 2003;44(12):1578–84.
18. Gilliam F, Kuzniecky R, Meador K, et al. Patient-oriented outcome assessment after temporal lobectomy for refractory epilepsy. Neurology 1999;53(4):687–94.
19. Fisher RS, Schachter SC. The postictal state: a neglected entity in the management of epilepsy. Epilepsy Behav 2000;1(1):52–9.
20. Blum DE, Eskola J, Bortz JJ, et al. Patient awareness of seizures. Neurology 1996; 47(1):260–4.
21. Heo K, Han SD, Lim SR, et al. Patient awareness of complex partial seizures. Epilepsia 2006;47(11):1931–5.
22. Poochikian-Sarkissian S, Tai P, del Campo M, et al. Patient awareness of seizures as documented in the epilepsy monitoring unit. Can J Neurosci Nurs 2009;31(4): 22–3.
23. Fisher RS. Tracking epilepsy with an electronic diary. Acta Paediatr 2010;99(4): 516–8.
24. Glueckauf RL, Girvin JP, Braun JR, et al. Consistency of seizure frequency estimates across time, methods, and observers. Health Psychol 1990;9(4): 427–34.
25. Neugebauer R. Reliability of seizure diaries in adult epileptic patients. Neuroepidemiology 1989;8(5):228–33.
26. Stone AA, Shiffman S, Schwartz JE, et al. Patient compliance with paper and electronic diaries. Control Clin Trials 2003;24(2):182–99.
27. Dale O, Hagen KB. Despite technical problems personal digital assistants outperform pen and paper when collecting patient diary data. J Clin Epidemiol 2007;60(1):8–17.
28. Le S, Shafer PO, Bartfeld E, et al. An online diary for tracking epilepsy. Epilepsy Behav 2011;22(4):705–9.
29. Conradsen I, Beniczky S, Wolf P, et al. Multi-modal intelligent seizure acquisition (MISA) system–a new approach towards seizure detection based on full body motion measures. Conf Proc IEEE Eng Med Biol Soc 2009;2009:2591–5.
30. Cuppens K, Lagae L, Ceulemans B, et al. Detection of nocturnal frontal lobe seizures in pediatric patients by means of accelerometers: a first study. Conf Proc IEEE Eng Med Biol Soc 2009;2009:6608–11.
31. Nijsen TM, Arends JB, Griep PA, et al. The potential value of three-dimensional accelerometry for detection of motor seizures in severe epilepsy. Epilepsy Behav 2005;7(1):74–84.
32. Carlson C, Arnedo V, Cahill M, et al. Detecting nocturnal convulsions: efficacy of the MP5 monitor. Seizure 2009;18(3):225–7.
33. Bayly J, Carino J, Petrovski S, et al. Time-frequency mapping of the rhythmic limb movements distinguishes convulsive epileptic from psychogenic nonepileptic seizures. Epilepsia 2013;54(8):1402–8.
34. Lockman J, Fisher RS, Olson DM. Detection of seizure-like movements using a wrist accelerometer. Epilepsy Behav 2011;20(4):638–41.
35. Kramer U, Kipervasser S, Shlitner A, et al. A novel portable seizure detection alarm system: preliminary results. J Clin Neurophysiol 2011;28(1):36–8.

36. Beniczky S, Polster T, Kjaer TW, et al. Detection of generalized tonic-clonic seizures by a wireless wrist accelerometer: a prospective, multicenter study. Epilepsia 2013;54(4):e58–61.
37. Velez M, Fisher RS, Bartlett V, et al. A biosensor for tracking seizures: linking a wrist accelerometer to an online epilepsy database. International League Against Epilepsy Congress. Istanbul (Turkey); September 8, 2015.
38. Conradsen I, Beniczky S, Hoppe K, et al. Seizure onset detection based on one sEMG channel. Conf Proc IEEE Eng Med Biol Soc 2011;2011:7715–8.
39. Larsen SN, Conradsen I, Beniczky S, et al. Detection of tonic epileptic seizures based on surface electromyography. Conf Proc IEEE Eng Med Biol Soc 2014; 2014:942–5.
40. Koss MC, Davison MA. Characteristics of the electrodermal response. A model for analysis of central sympathetic reactivity. Naunyn Schmiedebergs Arch Pharmacol 1976;295(2):153–8.
41. Sequeira H, Hot P, Silvert L, et al. Electrical autonomic correlates of emotion. Int J Psychophysiol 2009;71(1):50–6.
42. Fletcher RR, Tam S, Omojola O, et al. Wearable sensor platform and mobile application for use in cognitive behavioral therapy for drug addiction and PTSD. Conf Proc IEEE Eng Med Biol Soc 2011;2011:1802–5.
43. Christie MJ. Electrodermal activity and the stress response. A review. Acta Med Pol 1973;14(4):343–55.
44. Simpson CJ, Hyde CE. Electrodermal response as a monitor in electroconvulsive therapy. Br J Psychiatry 1987;150:549–51.
45. Turkstra LS. Electrodermal response and outcome from severe brain injury. Brain Inj 1995;9(1):61–80.
46. Daltrozzo J, Wioland N, Mutschler V, et al. Emotional electrodermal response in coma and other low-responsive patients. Neurosci Lett 2010;475(1):44–7.
47. Moseley BD. Seizure-related autonomic changes in children. J Clin Neurophysiol 2015;32(1):5–9.
48. Van Buren JM. Some autonomic concomitants of ictal automatism: a study of temporal lobe attacks. Brain 1958;81:505–28.
49. Fletcher RR, Dobson K, Goodwin MS, et al. iCalm: wearable sensor and network architecture for wirelessly communicating and logging autonomic activity. Conf Proc IEEE Eng Med Biol Soc 2010;14(2):215–23.
50. Poh MZ, Loddenkemper T, Swenson NC, et al. Continuous monitoring of electrodermal activity during epileptic seizures using a wearable sensor. Conf Proc IEEE Eng Med Biol Soc 2010;2010:4415–8.
51. Poh MZ, Swenson NC, Picard RW. A wearable sensor for unobtrusive, long-term assessment of electrodermal activity. IEEE Trans Biomed Eng 2010;57(5):1243–52.
52. Poh MZ, Loddenkemper T, Reinsberger C, et al. Autonomic changes with seizures correlate with postictal EEG suppression. Neurology 2012;78(23):1868–76.
53. Maganti RK, Rutecki P. EEG and epilepsy monitoring. Continuum (Minneap Minn) 2013;19(3 Epilepsy):598–622.
54. Ives JR. 4-channel 24 hour cassette recorder for long-term EEG monitoring of ambulatory patients. Electroencephalogr Clin Neurophysiol 1975;39(1):88–92.
55. Seneviratne U, Mohamed A, Cook M, et al. The utility of ambulatory electroencephalography in routine clinical practice: a critical review. Epilepsy Res 2013; 105(1–2):1–12.
56. Stefan H, Kreiselmeyer G, Kasper B, et al. Objective quantification of seizure frequency and treatment success via long-term outpatient video-EEG monitoring: a feasibility study. Seizure 2011;20(2):97–100.

57. Faulkner HJ, Arima H, Mohamed A. The utility of prolonged outpatient ambulatory EEG. Seizure 2012;21(7):491–5.

58. Grummett TS, Leibbrandt RE, Lewis TW, et al. Measurement of neural signals from inexpensive, wireless and dry EEG systems. Physiol Meas 2015;36(7): 1469–84.

59. Fiedler P, Pedrosa P, Griebel S, et al. Novel multipin electrode cap system for dry electroencephalography. Brain Topogr 2015;28(5):647–56.

60. Huang YJ, Wu CY, Wong AM, et al. Novel active comb-shaped dry electrode for EEG measurement in hairy site. IEEE Trans Biomed Eng 2015;62(1):256–63.

61. Lopez-Gordo MA, Sanchez-Morillo D, Pelayo Valle F. Dry EEG electrodes. Sensors (Basel) 2014;14(7):12847–70.

62. Dias NS, Carmo JP, Mendes PM, et al. Wireless instrumentation system based on dry electrodes for acquiring EEG signals. Med Eng Phys 2012;34(7):972–81.

63. Gargiulo G, Calvo RA, Bifulco P, et al. A new EEG recording system for passive dry electrodes. Clin Neurophysiol 2010;121(5):686–93.

64. Leleux P, Badier JM, Rivnay J, et al. Conducting polymer electrodes for electroencephalography. Adv Healthc Mater 2014;3(4):490–3.

65. Chen YH, Op de Beeck M, Vanderheyden L, et al. Soft, comfortable polymer dry electrodes for high quality ECG and EEG recording. Sensors (Basel) 2014; 14(12):23758–80.

66. Howbert JJ, Patterson EE, Stead SM, et al. Forecasting seizures in dogs with naturally occurring epilepsy. PLoS One 2014;9(1):e81920.

67. Kossoff EH, Ritzl EK, Politsky JM, et al. Effect of an external responsive neurostimulator on seizures and electrographic discharges during subdural electrode monitoring. Epilepsia 2004;45(12):1560–7.

68. Morrell M. Brain stimulation for epilepsy: can scheduled or responsive neurostimulation stop seizures? Curr Opin Neurol 2006;19(2):164–8.

69. Sun FT, Morrell MJ, Wharen RE Jr. Responsive cortical stimulation for the treatment of epilepsy. Neurotherapeutics 2008;5(1):68–74.

70. Skarpaas TL, Morrell MJ. Intracranial stimulation therapy for epilepsy. Neurotherapeutics 2009;6(2):238–43.

71. Sun FT, Morrell MJ. Closed-loop neurostimulation: the clinical experience. Neurotherapeutics 2014;11(3):553–63.

72. Morrell MJ, Group RNSSiES. Responsive cortical stimulation for the treatment of medically intractable partial epilepsy. Neurology 2011;77(13):1295–304.

73. King-Stephens D, Mirro E, Weber PB, et al. Lateralization of mesial temporal lobe epilepsy with chronic ambulatory electrocorticography. Epilepsia 2015;56(6): 959–67.

Assessment of Treatment Side Effects and Quality of Life in People with Epilepsy

Benjamin N. Blond, MD, Kamil Detyniecki, MD,
Lawrence J. Hirsch, MD*

KEYWORDS

- Epilepsy • Adverse medication effects • Quality of life • Structured assessment
- Depression

KEY POINTS

- Seizure freedom dramatically improves quality of life.
- When seizure freedom cannot be achieved, the effects of psychiatric comorbidities and medications have a larger impact on quality of life.
- Tools for structured assessment of quality of life and medication effects can improve the level of care.

INTRODUCTION

Quality of life (QOL) is a broad term encompassing not just the absence of disease, but an individual's perception of his or her position in life and goals, expectations, and concerns. People with epilepsy (PWE) face a condition that can affect their QOL in multiple domains. These include physical (seizures predict increased risk of injury and death), psychological (increased risk of anxiety and depression), cognitive (both epilepsy and the medications used to treat it are associated with impaired cognition), and social and occupational (epilepsy is a stigmatizing condition, and also often carries limitations on driving and employment). This review provides a concise discussion of the main determinants of QOL in epilepsy, various tools for the structured assessment of QOL, and some additional resources available to clinicians to improve the QOL of their patients. One of the areas in which clinicians can have the greatest impact is in the management of the side effects of antiepileptic drugs (AEDs), and thus assessment of medication adverse events is a particular focus. Mood disorders are discussed more thoroughly in a separate article [see Fiest KM, Patten SB, Jetté N: Screening for Depression and Anxiety in Epilepsy, in this issue].

Department of Neurology, Comprehensive Epilepsy Center, Yale University, New Haven, CT, USA
* Corresponding author. Yale Comprehensive Epilepsy Center, PO Box 208018, New Haven, CT 06520-8018.
E-mail address: lawrence.hirsch@yale.edu

Neurol Clin 34 (2016) 395–410
http://dx.doi.org/10.1016/j.ncl.2015.11.002
0733-8619/16/$ – see front matter © 2016 Elsevier Inc. All rights reserved.
neurologic.theclinics.com

MAIN DETERMINANTS OF QUALITY OF LIFE IN EPILEPSY
Seizures

Epilepsy is a condition defined by recurrent seizures and the presence of these seizures has a major impact on QOL. Studies that have included broadly applicable QOL scales have found that PWE who were seizure free had a QOL comparable to the general population, whereas individuals with seizures had impairments across multiple domains.[1,2] These impairments are clinically significant and can be severe. In one study comparing QOL in PWE who underwent epilepsy surgery with people with other chronic diseases, the presence of any seizures within the past year, even when these seizures did not impair consciousness, led to impaired QOL at a level comparable to patients with hypertension, diabetes, heart disease, or depressive symptoms, whereas PWE who were seizure free had superior QOL compared with all other groups.[3]

The exact relation between seizure frequency and QOL is complex. Many studies have suggested that in PWE with seizures, seizure frequency does not correlate with QOL, and that sustained improvements in QOL are only seen in individuals who are completely seizure free.[2–7] However, there also have been multiple studies that have demonstrated significant effects of seizure frequency on QOL.[1,8–14] The reason for these discrepant findings is likely related to variability between studies in areas such as the length of time required to be considered seizure free, the frequency of seizures in patients who are not seizure free, whether or not auras are included as seizures, the specific scales used to assess QOL, and the power of the studies to detect smaller effects. Despite this variability in the literature, some consistent themes emerge. In all of the previously mentioned studies, seizure freedom leads to dramatic improvements in QOL. Studies that did find a significant effect of seizure frequency on QOL noted more modest improvements than in individuals who were seizure free. To see an effect, the research generally required either rare seizures[9,13] or major reductions in seizures of at least 75%.[12,14] In patients with refractory epilepsy with multiple seizures each month, seizure frequency does not appear to influence QOL significantly.[5,6] Overall, for individuals for whom seizure freedom cannot be achieved, factors other than seizure frequency have a predominant impact on QOL.[10] These include mood and adverse effects of medications.

Psychiatric Comorbidities

Psychiatric comorbidities can have a profound impact on QOL in both neurologic and non-neurologic conditions. This is especially important in epilepsy where depression, anxiety, and suicidal ideation are at significantly increased prevalence compared with the general population.[15] Indeed, in refractory epilepsy, the prevalence of depression has been estimated to be as high as 50%.[16] Studies examining a range of cognitive functions and QOL have shown that depressed mood has the highest correlation with negative QOL, and can explain approximately 50% of the variance among subjects.[17,18] A large survey identified that patients with depression had significantly worsened QOL, and perceived greater seizure severity.[19] Depression has been found to be a major predictor of QOL across varying domains and of activities of daily living after controlling for seizure frequency.[20] Multiple studies have simultaneously examined the effects of both seizure frequency and depression on QOL. Although there has been significant variability in whether seizure frequency had a significant impact on QOL and to what degree, the research has consistently shown that depression and anxiety have a greater degree of association with QOL than seizure frequency in individuals who are not seizure free.[5,6,21,22] There has been less research on the impact of comorbid anxiety, but this too appears to have major implications for QOL in PWE. A recent study demonstrated that both depression and anxiety, although highly correlated with each other, were each independently associated with worsened QOL at all levels of seizure control.[9] For a more comprehensive discussion on depression and anxiety, please see [Fiest KM, Patten SB, Jetté N: Screening for Depression and Anxiety in Epilepsy, in this issue].

Antiepileptic Drug Effects

AEDs can have a major impact on QOL in PWE. Baker and colleagues[23] had more than 5000 PWE complete questionnaires on QOL. In their sample, only 12% of PWE reported no side effects from their medications and 31% reported changing medications at least once as a result of side effects. Adverse medication effects have been linked to worsened QOL[24,25] and institution of a structured assessment of AED side effects to clinic visits demonstrated reduction in side effects and improvements in QOL.[23] Given the importance of this topic and the level of control clinicians have in adjusting AEDs, the assessment of the effects of medications is discussed at greater length in the following sections.

Cognition

Cognitive impairments are highly associated with epilepsy and are often multifactorial. There is a component of inherent cognitive deficits related to the underlying brain pathology, but there are also more modifiable components attributed to the effects of seizure frequency and pattern, AEDs, and psychiatric comorbidities.[26] Whether poorly controlled seizures cause progressive deterioration of cognitive functions, and if so, how often, remains unclear.[27,28] In many types of epilepsy, cognitive impairments appear to be independent of seizure frequency, with evidence of these deficits preceding seizure onset and persisting despite seizure freedom. There is some evidence that recurrent seizures worsen cognitive outcome in mesial temporal lobe epilepsy and some of the epileptic encephalopathies, including West syndrome and epilepsy with continuous spike and wave during slow wave sleep. In these syndromes, seizure control may play an important role in preserving cognition and QOL, but outside of these limited situations, clinicians can focus on treating mood and medication side effects to improve QOL in relation to cognition.

Sleep

Sleep and epilepsy are highly interrelated.[29] Non–rapid eye movement sleep can activate interictal discharges and affect seizure threshold, and differing circadian rhythm abnormalities have been associated with different epilepsy syndromes. However, epilepsy may also have profound effects on sleep with evidence for alteration in sleep patterns and higher than expected prevalence of sleep apnea, periodic limb movements, restless leg syndrome, insomnia, hypersomnia, and parasomnias in children. AEDs may worsen this situation through a disruptive effect on sleep architecture. Studies have shown that the presence of a comorbid sleep disorder significantly worsens QOL in epilepsy.[30,31]

Migraine

PWE are more than twice as likely to have migraines than the general population.[32] This highly increased prevalence is in part explained by patients with head trauma as a cause of both conditions, but PWE without a history of head trauma also show an increased risk of migraine headaches. The effect of comorbid migraines on QOL in PWE has not been specifically evaluated, but migraine is known to cause impaired QOL in the general population[33] and is therefore important to diagnose and treat.

Social Impairments

Finally, there has been increasing recognition of the social impacts of epilepsy. Indeed, in a multicenter trial of patients with epilepsy who received surgery, patients who achieved seizure freedom had comparable QOL to the general population in all domains except social functioning, where they still faced impairments.[2] These impairments are likely multifactorial. PWE can have impaired social interaction due to the cognitive limitations they face in processing speed and attentional abilities. They face restrictions that can impair their participation in social activities, and can face significant stigma. There is also some work to suggest that specific social abilities, including theory of mind, are impaired in people with frontal and temporal lobe and idiopathic generalized epilepsy.[34] PWE demonstrate lower rates of marriage and employment and have fewer children. With this in mind, there is increasing development of programs to provide social support. For a detailed review of social functioning in epilepsy, see Szemere and Jokeit.[35]

METHODS OF ASSESSMENT OF QUALITY OF LIFE

Structured assessment of QOL in epilepsy is important both in the conduct of research and in the clinical evaluation of patients. Multiple questionnaires have been used in research on QOL in epilepsy, including more than 20 that are specific to epilepsy. However, some of these questionnaires have not been thoroughly validated, others have only been used sparingly, and some questionnaires lack an assessment of important areas, such as AED side effects. Several of the scales in use are highlighted later in this article and the test characteristics are reported in **Table 1**; for a more detailed review, see Jacoby and colleagues.[36]

The first scales used to assess QOL in epilepsy were generic measures used for multiple diseases. The SF-36[37] is a short-form health survey that looks at functioning in a variety of domains and has been used in research on QOL in epilepsy. This scale was used as a foundation for the creation of epilepsy-specific scales. The first scale to do so was the Epilepsy Surgery Inventory (ESI-55),[4] in which 19 questions were added to the SF-36 to address epilepsy-specific issues, including memory and cognitive function, with the goal of assessing QOL in PWE who underwent surgery. The Quality of Life in Epilepsy Scale (QOLIE)[38] was developed to be more expansive in scope both in including more patient populations and addressing more social limitations. It has been well validated and has become the most commonly used scale in the assessment of QOL in epilepsy. It has been shown to remain valid in administration via telephone and in translation to a number of different languages, both expanding the reach of the scale.

Some scales assessing QOL in epilepsy were developed to look at particular aspects of the disease. The Washington Psychosocial Inventory (WPSI)[39] was developed to specifically assess the psychosocial concerns of those with epilepsy. The Neurologic Disorders Depression Inventory for Epilepsy (NDDI-E) was developed to reliably and consistently diagnose depression in individuals with epilepsy. The very brief scale comprises only 6 items, and a score of 15 has an 81% sensitivity, 90% specificity, and is not confounded by the adverse effects of medications.[40]

The Liverpool QOL Batteries take a composite approach. The assessment is composed of multiple subscales that could be included according to different research questions or different clinical situations with the goal of tailored instruments leading to a superior assessment. The possible subscales include tools to assess seizure severity, AED effects, neuropsychological effects, impact on driving and independence, and the stigma PWE face. There is also a scale specifically designed to address individuals with new-onset epilepsy: NEWQOL.

Although essential for research, these comprehensive assessments are time-consuming. There have been multiple efforts to create tools that can be administered briefly without losing significant breadth and depth. The QOLIE-89 has been modified into versions with 31[41] and 10[42] questions, with the specific intention for the latter to be of practical clinical use. Most recently, Fisher and colleagues[43] developed the Personal Impact of Epilepsy Scale (PIES), using feedback from individuals with epilepsy in response to open-ended questions to create a patient-reported outcome instrument that has been found to correlate well with prior validated scales, including the Seizure Severity Scale, Liverpool Adverse Events Profile, and QOLIE-31.

ASSESSMENT OF MEDICATION EFFECTS

Despite recent advances in surgery and neurostimulation, the mainstay of therapy for epilepsy remains AEDs. The goal of AEDs is to achieve seizure control; however, this is often limited by toxicity. Although numerous new drugs exist to treat seizures, there is a lack of high-quality comparative data on their effectiveness. Clinicians often rely on other factors, such as adverse effect profile, familiarity, ease of use, and cost, rather than effectiveness to choose an AED. In a large survey of PWE conducted by the Epilepsy Foundation, only 68% of participants were satisfied with their current antiepileptic medication. When asked to rank important features of their AEDs, adverse reaction was ranked second after seizure control.[44] Adverse effects of AEDs impair QOL as noted previously. They also have a significant effect on morbidity and can contribute to increased health care utilization and costs directly, or indirectly due to failed therapy and poor adherence.

Identifying side effects in an outpatient clinic can be challenging due to confounding factors, time constraints, and a lack of a standard nomenclature. Patients may use terms like dizziness, vertigo, and lightheadedness as synonyms. Also, patients may report memory complaints when in fact they are experiencing anomia or depression. Establishing cause-effect is often difficult and patients may interpret symptoms related to their epilepsy, such as the migraines and cognitive and mood impairments discussed previously, as an adverse effect of their medication instead.

Communication of medication adverse events to regulatory agencies occurs during drug development and after marketing. The incidence of common adverse effects is based on patient self-report. This requires the use of standard medical terminology that translates the colloquial language of patient reports of side effects into an internationally accepted coding system, which could aid in the transmission and translation of reports from various parts of the world.

The World Health Organization's (WHO's) definition of an adverse drug reaction is "a response to a drug that is noxious and unintended and occurs at doses normally used in man for the prophylaxis, diagnosis or therapy of disease, or for modification of physiologic function."[45] Adverse drug effects can be classified according to their mechanism of action, organ or structure affected, frequency, and severity. There have been several attempts to unify adverse effect terminology so that drugs could be easily compared.

The WHO Adverse Reaction Terminology (WHO-ART) has been used by regulatory agencies and pharmaceutical manufacturers alongside the International Classification of Diseases for more than 30 years to rationally code clinical information related to adverse drug reactions. WHO-ART is a 4-level hierarchical terminology, which begins

Table 1
Scales for assessment of QOL in PWE

Scale Name	Description	Contents	Estimated Time to Completion	Advantages	Disadvantages
SF-36[37]	Short-form health survey	36 questions on physical functioning (10), role limitations due to physical functions (4), social functioning (2), bodily pain (2), general mental health (5), role limitations due to emotional problems (3), vitality (4), general health perceptions (5)	5–10 min	Generic core of later epilepsy-specific measures. Allows for comparison with other medical conditions.	Not specific to epilepsy.
Washington Psychosocial Inventory (WPSI)[39]	Assesses the psychosocial concerns of adults with epilepsy	132 items addressing the following 8 subscales: family background, emotional, interpersonal, vocational adjustment, financial status, adjustment to seizures, medical management, ad overall functioning	15–20 min	Good psychometric properties.	Does not address physical functioning, energy, and cognition.
Epilepsy Surgery Inventory (ESI-55)[4]	Designed to assess QOL in people who had surgery for intractable epilepsy	Health perceptions (9); energy/fatigue (4); overall QOL (2); social function (2); emotional well-being (5); cognitive function (5); physical function (10); pain (2); role limitations due to physical, emotional, or memory problems (5 each); change in health (1)	15 min	Good psychometric properties.	Excess ceiling effect.

Scale	Purpose	Description	Time	Advantages	Disadvantages
Quality of Life in Epilepsy Scales (QOLIE-89, 31, and 10)[38,41,42]	Assess QOL in PWE	89-question scale covering 17 different sections evaluating both general and epilepsy-specific QOL, including areas such as seizure worry, AED effects, cognition, social limitations, limitations in work and driving, and health discouragement	89-item version: 15–25 min; 31-item version: 5–15 min; 10-item version: "several min"	Extensively validated, available in different languages, can be administered by phone, ability to discriminate between QOL among patients with different seizure frequencies.	—
Liverpool HRQOL Batteries[36]	Assesses the effects of epilepsy on physical, social, and psychological function	Various combinations of multiple different subscales	30–40 min depending on combination used	Battery allows tailoring the subscales to the particular clinical situation or research question.	Time-consuming to complete.
Personal Impact of Epilepsy Scale (PIES)[43]	Recently developed patient-reported outcome measure for epilepsy	25 questions: seizure characteristics (9), medication side effects (7), comorbidities (8), quality of life (1)	5–10 min	Brief, developed using patient-generated concerns regarding QOL.	New, not yet tested for sensitivity to change in therapies or patient condition.

Abbreviations: AED, antiepileptic drug; HRQOL, health-related quality of life; PWE, people with epilepsy; QOL, quality of life.

at the body system/organ-level classes. These classes consist of broad grouping terms, which in turn consist of more specific preferred terms.

Another coding system that was previously used by the US Food and Drug Administration (FDA) is *The Coding Symbols for a Thesaurus of Adverse Reaction Terms* (COSTART). COSTART is organized in body system and pathophysiology hierarchies, as well as a separate fetal/neonatal category.

These terminologies have been criticized for lack of specificity, limited data retrieval options, and an inability to effectively handle complex combinations of signs and symptoms (syndromes). There is also concern for obscuring valuable safety signals by lumping and splitting terms. In addition, pharmaceutical companies may use different terminologies at different stages in the drug development and use of products, which complicates data retrieval and analysis of information.

Given this need for standardized medical terminology, the International Conference on Harmonization developed *The Medical Dictionary for Regulatory Activities* (MedDRA) using input from regulatory agencies and pharmaceutical companies. MedDRA is a hierarchical system composed of various levels of terminology (ie, system organ class, high-level group term, high-level term, preferred term, lower-level term). The preferred term provides medically validated representations of colloquial terms, which could result in fewer misrepresentations and misunderstandings of colloquial reports from various parts of the world. Its use is currently mandated in Europe and Japan for safety reporting. MedDRA is not currently required at the FDA; however, most drug reports from manufacturers are received electronically, precoded in MedDRA.

In addition to coding and terminology difficulties, reporting of side effects can be biased by patients' and physicians' expectations. For example, in clinical trials, higher rates of rash were seen in the placebo group when the active drug was lamotrigine.[46] Similarly, one may expect higher rates of irritability reported in patients taking levetiracetam when they were warned about that particular side effect previously.

Assessing adverse effects based on patient spontaneous self-report has been used and continues to be a common form of reporting side effects in clinical practice and clinical trials. However, this may lead to underreporting, as studies using structured interviews or questionnaires report a higher rate of adverse effects for the same drugs compared with patient self-report.[46,47] In the next section, we discuss the use of valid and reliable instruments to assess medication side effects.

STRUCTURED ASSESSMENT OF SIDE EFFECTS

Several validated instruments exist to assess medication side effects in PWE. Most consist of a list of common complaints or questions using colloquial language that was developed based on patients' spontaneous reports and from observations and input from leaders in the field. These simple tools have been validated in several studies and have good psychometric properties, including reliability and responsiveness necessary for their use in research and clinical settings. **Table 2** displays the most commonly used scales in epilepsy.

The scales or questionnaires are usually completed by the patients. Patients answer using a Likert scale rating the frequency or severity of occurring symptoms in the previous weeks. In the case of pediatric scales, parents grade the symptoms.[48,49] An exception is the Department of Veterans Affairs systemic and neurotoxicity scale, in which assessment is obtained based on direct questioning by the treating physician and examination/direct observation of potential problems, such as rash, gait, and so forth.[50] All toxicity is compared with normal for each patient before starting the medication.

Table 2
Common tools used in patients with epilepsy to assess medication side effects

Scale Name	Administration	Scope of Side Effects Reviewed	Structure/Scoring System	Estimated Time to Complete, min	Advantages	Disadvantages
VA systemic and neurotoxicity scales[50]	Physician-administered Questioning followed by examination of symptoms	Systemic, neurotoxic, and seizures frequency rating.	Systemic toxicity Score (8 questions). Neurotoxicity score (8 questions). Composite score (summation of scores + seizure frequency rating). Rating based on frequency and severity of symptoms.	20	Includes direct evaluation and confirmation by physician of the side effects. Includes sexual side effects, abnormal laboratory findings, rash.	Does not include sleep disturbances, hair loss. Complex scoring system Time-consuming.
Adverse Event Profile (AEP)[23]	Self-administered	Systemic and neurologic.	19 items (symptoms). Rating based on frequency. Scores for each symptom and composite score.	5–10	Good psychometric properties. Validated in several studies. Available in several languages.	Many symptoms listed as possible effects of AEDs are also symptoms of anxiety and depression. Does not include sexual side effects.
Side-effects in AED treatment (SIAED)[51]	Self-administered	10 categories: general CNS, behavior, depressive symptoms, cognitive function, motor problems, visual complaints, headache, cosmetic, gastrointestinal, sexuality, and menses	46 items. Rating based on severity and duration.	10	Includes a comprehensive list of complaints, such as sleep, sexuality, and menses.	Its psychometric properties have not been well validated.

(continued on next page)

Table 2
(continued)

Scale Name	Administration	Scope of Side Effects Reviewed	Structure/Scoring System	Estimated Time to Complete, min	Advantages	Disadvantages
A-B Neuro psychological Assessment Scale (ABNAS)[52]	Self-administered	Cognitive adverse events. Covers areas such as fatigue, slowing, hyperexcitability, memory, concentration, motor coordination and language.	24 items. Rating based on severity.	5	Very sensitive at detecting impairments.	Results on the scale cannot be used to draw conclusions about impairment in specific cognitive domains. Does not take into account the mood of the patient.
Portland Neurotoxicity Scale (PNS)[53]	Self-administered	Neurotoxic symptoms (mainly cognitive difficulties, lack of coordination and blurry vision).	15 items. Rating based on severity.	5	Good psychometric properties and sensitive to AED usage in test-retest studies.	—
The Side-Effect and Life Satisfaction scale (SEALS)[56]	Self-administered	Psychosocial effects of AED therapy. 5 subscales: worry, temper, cognition, dysphoria, tiredness.	38 questions related to the patient's feelings and behavior. Rating based on frequency. Individual scores for each factor and an overall score.	5–10	Includes psychosocial effects. Good psychometric properties. Translated into several languages. Sensitive to small change in HRQOL.	—

Instrument	Administration	Description	Items/Rating	Duration	Advantages	Limitations
Epworth Sleepiness Screening scale (ESS)[54]	Self-administered	Sleepiness in 8 different situations (such as watching TV or sitting and reading).	8 items. Rating based on the likelihood of dozing off or falling asleep in each of the situations.	<5 min	Simple and short duration.	Sleepiness can be multifactorial. Does not distinguish AED SE from symptoms of OSA and RLS.
American Urologic Association Index System (AUA SI)[55]	Self-administered	Urologic symptoms (frequency, nocturia, weak urinary stream, hesitancy, intermittence, incomplete emptying and urgency).	7 questions. Rating based on severity.	5	Good at measuring changes in symptom severity over time.	Unable to discriminate symptoms from primary urologic disorders, such as BPH vs AED SE.
The Hague Side-Effect Scale (HASES)[49] PEDIATRIC	Parent report	Toxic (dose dependent) and long-term behavioral and cognitive side effects.	20 items. Rating based on severity. 2 subscales: toxic subscale, chronic subscale.	5	Includes acute and chronic side effects. Includes school performance as a measure.	Some terms used are vague and may be inconsistently reported, whereas others may be used interchangeably.
Pediatric Epilepsy Side-Effects Questionnaire (PESQ)[48] PEDIATRIC	Parent report Self-administered (adolescents)	5 categories: cognitive, motor, behavioral, general neurologic, and weight.	19 items. Rating based on severity. 5 subscales.	5	Includes weight. Uses common colloquial language.	Does not include rare side effects such as severe rash or kidney stones.

Abbreviations: AED, antiepileptic drug; BPH, benign prostatic hyperplasia; CNS, central nervous system; OSA, obstructive sleep apnea; RLS, restless leg syndrome; SE, side effect; VA, Department of Veterans Affairs.

The scope of these scales varies. Some include general systemic and neurologic complaints that are grouped into categories, such as in the Adverse Event Profile (AEP)[23] and in Side-effects in AED treatment (SIAED).[51] Others, such as the A-B Neuropsychological Assessment Scale (ABNAS)[52] or the Portland Neurotoxicity Scale (PNS),[53] concentrate on neurotoxic symptoms, mainly cognitive difficulties, especially concentration and memory.

There are also specific scales that were initially developed to assess symptoms of other conditions that have been found to be useful screening tools in PWE. This is the case of the Epworth Sleepiness Scale (ESS),[54] which was developed to monitor the propensity of falling asleep in patients with sleep disorders such as obstructive sleep apnea or narcolepsy. Similarly, the American Urologic Association Index System (UAA SI),[55] developed to monitor symptoms of benign prostatic hyperplasia, can be useful in assessing urologic symptoms in PWE taking ezogabine.

Some scales have attempted to look at psychosocial effects of AED therapy and impact on QOL, including SIAED and the Side Effect and Life Satisfaction (SEALS) inventory.[56] SEALS scores are sensitive to small changes in QOL.[57,58] However, caution is advised when interpreting the results of these assessment tools. Other factors, such as depression and anxiety may influence the results. In a cohort of newly diagnosed PWE, anxiety scores were the major predictors of global AEP scores,[59] and as noted previously, this may be directly associated with epilepsy and not the AEDs.

SELF-MANAGEMENT STRATEGIES TO IMPROVE QUALITY OF LIFE

Research on assessment of QOL in epilepsy is increasingly focusing on the resilience of PWE, as fostering this trait can lead to improvements in QOL.[60] Along these lines, some researchers have investigated structured systems in which PWE can better manage their conditions. Several programs have been developed to provide educational and/or psychosocial support, with promising results, although the small sample size of most studies limits firm conclusions.

Some interventions consist of brief educational programs. One early study found that a 2-day educational program for patients and caregivers led to increased epilepsy knowledge, decreased fear of seizures, reduction in hazardous self-management of medications, and decreased information misunderstanding.[61] The study also demonstrated increased medication compliance, as corroborated by a 70% increase in serum AED levels in the treatment group, compared with an 18% decrease in serum AED levels in the control group. Another 2-day course, MOSES (Modular Service Package Epilepsy), provides education on epilepsy, including epidemiology, diagnosis, and treatment to patients, as well as covering the psychosocial aspects of the condition. This has demonstrated benefit in randomized controlled trials in improving knowledge about epilepsy and coping strategies, although the currently limited data fail to show a significant improvement in QOL.[62] The Self-Management education for adults with poorly controlled epilepsy (SMILE UK) trial aims to improve knowledge in this area, by recruiting approximately 400 subjects into a randomized controlled trial using a version of MOSES adapted for the United Kingdom.[63]

Programs focusing on psychosocial concerns have tended to have more longitudinal structures. PACES is a group-based psycho educational intervention that was developed with the input of individuals with epilepsy.[64] The program consisted of 8 weekly 75-minute sessions as part of a randomized unblinded trial. The intervention group demonstrated improvements in several areas of QOL, including QOLIE-31, at the completion of the program, and there was some sustained benefit of the program

Table 3	
Managing epilepsy well network web programs	
Web Epilepsy Awareness Support and Education (WebEase)	Interactive program that aims to address medication adherence, stress reduction, and sleep management. It helps users create goals for self-management and track their progress.
Using Practice and Learning to Increase Favorable Thoughts (UPLIFT)—Treatment	Uses 8 weekly sessions of mindfulness-based cognitive therapy to help treat depression in groups of 6–8 by telephone or Internet, facilitated by a graduate student in mental health and a PWE.
Using Practice and Learning to Increase Favorable Thoughts (UPLIFT)— Prevention	An adaptation of the treatment program aimed at prevention of depression in PWE identified as at risk.
Management Information Decision Support Epilepsy Tool (MINDSET)	Tablet-based program aimed at providing real-time decision support to patients and providers in the context of an epilepsy clinic visit.
Program to Encourage Active Rewarding Lives for Seniors (PEARLS)	A home-based depression treatment program involving problem solving, behavioral activation, and psychiatric consultation. The Web-based program is intended for professionals interested in implementing PEARLS in their local communities.

Adapted from Shegog R, Bamps YA, Patel A, et al. Managing epilepsy well: emerging e-Tools for epilepsy self-management. Epilepsy Behav 2013;29(1):133–40.

at reassessment 6 months later in information management, energy and fatigue, and medication side-effects measures.

As educational and psychosocial interventions have shown promise, there has been increasing interest in how best to deliver these interventions to expand access and benefit. The Managing Epilepsy Well Network has developed a number of Web-based applications designed to assist in epilepsy self-management, as detailed in **Table 3**. WebEase demonstrated an increase in self-reported medication adherence and self-efficacy in a randomized trial.[65]

SUMMARY

Epilepsy is a condition with a profound impact on QOL, with often severe levels of impairment across physical, cognitive, emotional, and social domains. The goal of treatment for PWE should always be seizure freedom, but when this cannot be achieved, other factors, particularly depression and adverse medication effects, can have a larger impact on QOL. Therefore, the screening for comorbid conditions and psychosocial effects is of paramount importance in maximizing the QOL of PWE. Structured assessments of QOL and medication effects are helpful in identifying such factors. Aggressive modification of identified impairments and potentially the use of self-management programs can help to improve QOL in PWE.

REFERENCES

1. Leidy NK, Elixhauser A, Vickrey B, et al. Seizure frequency and the health-related quality of life of adults with epilepsy. Neurology 1999;53(1):162–6.

2. Spencer SS, Berg AT, Vickrey BG, et al. Health-related quality of life over time since resective epilepsy surgery. Ann Neurol 2007;62(4):327–34.

3. Vickrey BG, Hays RD, Rausch R, et al. Quality of life of epilepsy surgery patients as compared with outpatients with hypertension, diabetes, heart disease, and/or depressive symptoms. Epilepsia 1994;35(3):597–607.

4. Vickrey BG, Hays RD, Graber J, et al. A health-related quality of life instrument for patients evaluated for epilepsy surgery. Med Care 1992;30(4):299–319.

5. Boylan LS, Flint LA, Labovitz DL, et al. Depression but not seizure frequency predicts quality of life in treatment-resistant epilepsy. Neurology 2004;62(2):258–61.

6. Luoni C, Bisulli F, Canevini MP, et al. Determinants of health-related quality of life in pharmacoresistant epilepsy: results from a large multicenter study of consecutively enrolled patients using validated quantitative assessments. Epilepsia 2011;52(12):2181–91.

7. Markand ON, Salanova V, Whelihan E, et al. Health-related quality of life outcome in medically refractory epilepsy treated with anterior temporal lobectomy. Epilepsia 2000;41(6):749–59.

8. Birbeck GL, Hays RD, Cui X, et al. Seizure reduction and quality of life improvements in people with epilepsy. Epilepsia 2002;43(5):535–8.

9. Hamid H, Blackmon K, Cong X, et al. Mood, anxiety, and incomplete seizure control affect quality of life after epilepsy surgery. Neurology 2014;82(10):887–94.

10. Elsharkawy AE, Thorbecke R, Ebner A, et al. Determinants of quality of life in patients with refractory focal epilepsy who were not eligible for surgery or who rejected surgery. Epilepsy Behav 2012;24(2):249–55.

11. Lowe AJ, David E, Kilpatrick CJ, et al. Epilepsy surgery for pathologically proven hippocampal sclerosis provides long-term seizure control and improved quality of life. Epilepsia 2004;45(3):237–42.

12. McLachlan RS, Rose KJ, Derry PA, et al. Health-related quality of life and seizure control in temporal lobe epilepsy. Ann Neurol 1997;41(4):482–9.

13. Kellett MW, Smith DF, Baker GA, et al. Quality of life after epilepsy surgery. J Neurol Neurosurg Psychiatry 1997;63(1):52–8.

14. Malmgren K, Sullivan M, Ekstedt G, et al. Health-related quality of life after epilepsy surgery: a Swedish multicenter study. Epilepsia 1997;38(7):830–8.

15. Tellez-Zenteno JF, Patten SB, Jette N, et al. Psychiatric comorbidity in epilepsy: a population-based analysis. Epilepsia 2007;48(12):2336–44.

16. Altshuler L, Rausch R, Delrahim S, et al. Temporal lobe epilepsy, temporal lobectomy, and major depression. J Neuropsychiatry Clin Neurosci 1999;11(4):436–43.

17. Perrine K, Hermann BP, Meador KJ, et al. The relationship of neuropsychological functioning to quality of life in epilepsy. Arch Neurol 1995;52(10):997–1003.

18. Loring DW, Meador KJ, Lee GP. Determinants of quality of life in epilepsy. Epilepsy Behav 2004;5(6):976–80.

19. Cramer JA, Blum D, Reed M, et al. The influence of comorbid depression on seizure severity. Epilepsia 2003;44(12):1578–84.

20. Lehrner J, Kalchmayr R, Serles W, et al. Health-related quality of life (HRQOL), activity of daily living (ADL) and depressive mood disorder in temporal lobe epilepsy patients. Seizure 1999;8(2):88–92.

21. Johnson EK, Jones JE, Seidenberg M, et al. The relative impact of anxiety, depression, and clinical seizure features on health-related quality of life in epilepsy. Epilepsia 2004;45(5):544–50.

22. Tracy JI, Dechant V, Sperling MR, et al. The association of mood with quality of life ratings in epilepsy. Neurology 2007;68(14):1101–7.

23. Baker GA, Jacoby A, Buck D, et al. Quality of life of people with epilepsy: a European study. Epilepsia 1997;38(3):353–62.
24. Gilliam F. Optimizing health outcomes in active epilepsy. Neurology 2002;58(8 Suppl 5):S9–20.
25. Sillanpaa M, Haataja L, Shinnar S. Perceived impact of childhood-onset epilepsy on quality of life as an adult. Epilepsia 2004;45(8):971–7.
26. Mula M, Cock HR. More than seizures: improving the lives of people with refractory epilepsy. Eur J Neurol 2015;22(1):24–30.
27. Avanzini G, Depaulis A, Tassinari A, et al. Do seizures and epileptic activity worsen epilepsy and deteriorate cognitive function? Epilepsia 2013;54(Suppl 8):14–21.
28. Laxer KD, Trinka E, Hirsch LJ, et al. The consequences of refractory epilepsy and its treatment. Epilepsy Behav 2014;37:59–70.
29. Jain SV, Kothare SV. Sleep and epilepsy. Semin Pediatr Neurol 2015;22(2):86–92.
30. de Weerd A, de Haas S, Otte A, et al. Subjective sleep disturbance in patients with partial epilepsy: a questionnaire-based study on prevalence and impact on quality of life. Epilepsia 2004;45(11):1397–404.
31. Piperidou C, Karlovasitou A, Triantafyllou N, et al. Influence of sleep disturbance on quality of life of patients with epilepsy. Seizure 2008;17(7):588–94.
32. Ottman R, Lipton RB. Comorbidity of migraine and epilepsy. Neurology 1994;44(11):2105–10.
33. Abu Bakar N, Tanprawate S, Lambru G, et al. Quality of life in primary headache disorders: a review. Cephalalgia 2015. [Epub ahead of print].
34. Giovagnoli AR, Franceschetti S, Reati F, et al. Theory of mind in frontal and temporal lobe epilepsy: cognitive and neural aspects. Epilepsia 2011;52(11):1995–2002.
35. Szemere E, Jokeit H. Quality of life is social–towards an improvement of social abilities in patients with epilepsy. Seizure 2015;26:12–21.
36. Jacoby A, Baker GA, Crossley J, et al. Tools for assessing quality of life in epilepsy patients. Expert Rev Neurother 2013;13(12):1355–69.
37. Ware JE Jr, Sherbourne CD. The MOS 36-item short-form health survey (SF-36). I. Conceptual framework and item selection. Med Care 1992;30(6):473–83.
38. Devinsky O, Vickrey BG, Cramer J, et al. Development of the quality of life in epilepsy inventory. Epilepsia 1995;36(11):1089–104.
39. Dodrill CB, Batzel LW, Queisser HR, et al. An objective method for the assessment of psychological and social problems among epileptics. Epilepsia 1980;21(2):123–35.
40. Gilliam FG, Barry JJ, Hermann BP, et al. Rapid detection of major depression in epilepsy: a multicentre study. Lancet Neurol 2006;5(5):399–405.
41. Cramer JA, Perrine K, Devinsky O, et al. Development and cross-cultural translations of a 31-item quality of life in epilepsy inventory. Epilepsia 1998;39(1):81–8.
42. Cramer JA, Perrine K, Devinsky O, et al. A brief questionnaire to screen for quality of life in epilepsy: the QOLIE-10. Epilepsia 1996;37(6):577–82.
43. Fisher RS, Nune G, Roberts SE, et al. The personal impact of epilepsy scale (PIES). Epilepsy Behav 2015;42:140–6.
44. Fisher RS, Vickrey BG, Gibson P, et al. The impact of epilepsy from the patient's perspective II: views about therapy and health care. Epilepsy Res 2000;41(1):53–61.
45. International drug monitoring: the role of national centres. Report of a WHO meeting. World Health Organ Tech Rep Ser 1972;498:1–25.

46. Cramer JA, Fisher R, Ben-Menachem E, et al. New antiepileptic drugs: comparison of key clinical trials. Epilepsia 1999;40(5):590–600.

47. Gilliam FG, Fessler AJ, Baker G, et al. Systematic screening allows reduction of adverse antiepileptic drug effects: a randomized trial. Neurology 2004;62(1):23–7.

48. Morita DA, Glauser TA, Modi AC. Development and validation of the Pediatric Epilepsy Side Effects Questionnaire. Neurology 2012;79(12):1252–8.

49. Carpay HA, Arts WF, Vermeulen J, et al. Parent-completed scales for measuring seizure severity and severity of side-effects of antiepileptic drugs in childhood epilepsy: development and psychometric analysis. Epilepsy Res 1996;24(3): 173–81.

50. Cramer JA, Smith DB, Mattson RH, et al. A method of quantification for the evaluation of antiepileptic drug therapy. Neurology 1983;33(3 Suppl 1):26–37.

51. Uijl SG, Uiterwaal CS, Aldenkamp AP, et al. A cross-sectional study of subjective complaints in patients with epilepsy who seem to be well-controlled with antiepileptic drugs. Seizure 2006;15(4):242–8.

52. Aldenkamp AP, Baker G, Pieters MS, et al. The Neurotoxicity Scale: the validity of a patient-based scale, assessing neurotoxicity. Epilepsy Res 1995;20(3): 229–39.

53. Salinsky MC, Storzbach D. The Portland Neurotoxicity Scale: validation of a brief self-report measure of antiepileptic-drug-related neurotoxicity. Assessment 2005; 12(1):107–17.

54. Johns MW. A new method for measuring daytime sleepiness: the Epworth sleepiness scale. Sleep 1991;14(6):540–5.

55. Barry MJ, Fowler FJ Jr, O'Leary MP, et al. The American Urological Association symptom index for benign prostatic hyperplasia. The Measurement Committee of the American Urological Association. J Urol 1992;148(5):1549–57 [discussion: 1564].

56. Gillham R, Bryant-Comstock L, Kane K. Validation of the side effect and life satisfaction (SEALS) inventory. Seizure 2000;9(7):458–63.

57. Brodie MJ, Richens A, Yuen AW. Double-blind comparison of lamotrigine and carbamazepine in newly diagnosed epilepsy. UK Lamotrigine/Carbamazepine monotherapy trial group. Lancet 1995;345(8948):476–9.

58. Steiner TJ, Dellaportas CI, Findley LJ, et al. Lamotrigine monotherapy in newly diagnosed untreated epilepsy: a double-blind comparison with phenytoin. Epilepsia 1999;40(5):601–7.

59. Panelli RJ, Kilpatrick C, Moore SM, et al. The Liverpool adverse events profile: relation to AED use and mood. Epilepsia 2007;48(3):456–63.

60. Edward KL, Cook M, Giandinoto JA. An integrative review of the benefits of self-management interventions for adults with epilepsy. Epilepsy Behav 2015;45: 195–204.

61. Helgeson DC, Mittan R, Tan SY, et al. Sepulveda epilepsy education: the efficacy of a psychoeducational treatment program in treating medical and psychosocial aspects of epilepsy. Epilepsia 1990;31(1):75–82.

62. Ried S, Specht U, Thorbecke R, et al. MOSES: an educational program for patients with epilepsy and their relatives. Epilepsia 2001;42(Suppl 3):76–80.

63. Kralj-Hans I, Goldstein LH, Noble AJ, et al. Self-Management education for adults with poorly controlled epILEpsy (SMILE (UK)): a randomised controlled trial protocol. BMC Neurol 2014;14:69.

64. Fraser RT, Johnson EK, Lashley S, et al. PACES in epilepsy: results of a self-management randomized controlled trial. Epilepsia 2015;56(8):1264–74.

65. Shegog R, Bamps YA, Patel A, et al. Managing epilepsy well: emerging e-Tools for epilepsy self-management. Epilepsy Behav 2013;29(1):133–40.

Issues for Women with Epilepsy

Naymeé J. Vélez-Ruiz, MD[a],*, Page B. Pennell, MD[b,c]

KEYWORDS

- Women • Epilepsy • Catamenial • Pregnancy • Antiepileptic drugs • Contraception

KEY POINTS

- Women with epilepsy may experience seizure patterns related to the menstrual cycle and are at risk of reproductive abnormalities and pregnancy complications.
- There are bidirectional pharmacokinetic interactions between antiepileptic drugs (AEDs) and hormonal contraceptives, which may result in reduced efficacy of either one.
- AED treatment during pregnancy is a balancing act between teratogenic risks to the fetus and maintaining maternal seizure control.
- Folic acid supplementation prior to and during pregnancy has been associated with a risk reduction in the occurrence of congenital malformations and cognitive teratogenesis.
- Estimates of AED exposure from breast milk suggest that it is low for many AEDs.

INTRODUCTION

Epilepsy is one of the most common chronic conditions affecting women. Although the prevalence of epilepsy and treatment approaches are similar for women and men, women are more likely to experience seizure patterns related to hormonal cycles and are at risk of reproductive alterations and pregnancy complications.

NEUROSTEROIDS

Neurosteroids are molecules that modulate brain excitability and, therefore, can affect the occurrence of seizures. Estrogen and progesterone, the primary reproductive

Preparation of this article was supported in part by NIH NINDS #2U01-NS038455 (N.J. Vélez-Ruiz and P.B. Pennell).

Conflicts of Interest: The authors have no conflicts of interest that are directly relevant to the content of this review.

[a] Division of Epilepsy, Department of Neurology, University of Miami, 1120 Northwest, 14th Street, Suite 1329, Miami, FL 33136, USA; [b] Division of Epilepsy, Department of Neurology, Brigham and Women's Hospital, Harvard Medical School, Harvard University, 75 Francis Street, Boston, MA 02115, USA; [c] Division of Women's Health, Brigham and Women's Hospital, Harvard Medical School, Harvard University, 75 Francis Street, Boston, MA 02115, USA
* Corresponding author.
E-mail address: nxv146@med.miami.edu

hormones for women, both affect neuronal excitability. The actions of neurosteroids on neuroexcitability occur via 2 mechanisms. The first is a short latency, nongenomic effect mediated by the neuronal membrane.[1,2] The second is a long-latency (hours to days) genomic effect.[2,3] Estrogen has been suggested as neuroexcitatory, and some women with epilepsy might be susceptible to its proconvulsant effect.[2] Progesterone, on the other hand, promotes neuroinhibition, primarily through the action of its metabolite, allopregnanolone, which acts as a positive allosteric modulator of γ-aminobutyric acid conductance.[2,4,5]

SEX STEROID HORMONE AXIS

Release of female reproductive steroid hormones is controlled by the hypothalamic-pituitary-ovarian axis through a bidirectional feedback loop, as shown in **Fig. 1**.[6] Gonadotropin-releasing hormone (GnRH) is secreted by the hypothalamus and stimulates release of follicle-stimulating hormone (FSH) by the pituitary. FSH stimulates formation of the ovarian follicles, which secrete estradiol (the main estrogen in women). Midcycle, a surge of luteinizing hormone (LH) induces oocyte maturation, ovulation, and conversion of the follicle into the corpus luteum. This marks the end of the follicular phase and the beginning of the luteal phase. After ovulation, the corpus luteum secretes progesterone. Progesterone inhibits secretion of GnRH, FSH, and LH. If there is no pregnancy, the corpus luteum regresses and production of progesterone and estradiol declines. When progesterone secretion tapers off and GnRH inhibition decreases, the cycle repeats.

CATAMENIAL EPILEPSY

The pattern of seizure clustering during certain parts of the menstrual cycle is termed catamenial, derived from the Greek, katamenios, meaning monthly.[2] The reported prevalence of catamenial epilepsy depends on the specific definition used during quantification. Menstrual seizure exacerbations have been reported in up to 70% of women with epilepsy, although a more strict definition used by Herzog and colleagues[7] in their 1997 study suggested that this pattern was present in approximately one-third of women with epilepsy.

Menstrual Cycle

The average menstrual cycle is 28 (24–35) days, with day 1 the first day of menses and ovulation occurring on day 14 (or day −14 to adjust for cycle lengths other than

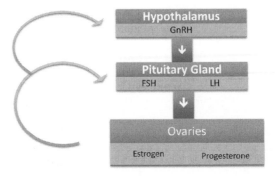

Fig. 1. Hypothalamic-pituitary-ovarian axis.

28 days, because ovulation always occurs 14 days prior to menses). The follicular phase then occurs during days 1 to 14 and the luteal phase on days 15 to 28 (or days −14 to −1). The hormonal fluctuations most relevant for catamenial seizure exacerbations are the rapid surge of estrogen at day 13, which initiates ovulation, and the rapid decline of progesterone followed by estrogen on days 26 to 28, just before the onset of menses.[2]

Dysregulated secretion of FSH leads to poor follicular development and, therefore, poor functioning of the corpus luteum. This disorder is known as inadequate luteal phase and is associated with lack of ovulation.[2,8] Inadequate development of the corpus luteum leads to low production of progesterone during the luteal phase, whereas estrogen production remains robust.[2]

Criteria for Diagnosis

The most accepted definition of catamenial epilepsy is based on the work of Herzog and colleagues,[7] who statistically derived the patterns of seizure occurrence throughout the menstrual cycle. They described an approximate doubling of seizure frequency during 3 portions of the menstrual cycle: perimenstrual (C1: days −3 to 3) and periovulatory (C2: days 10 to −13) in normal cycles and luteal (C3: days 10 to 3) in inadequate luteal phase cycles.[9] In the National Institutes of Health (NIH) Progesterone Treatment Trial, the prevalence of catamenial epilepsy by pattern was 39.8% C1, 33.9% C2, and 47.1% C3.[10] **Table 1** shows each type with its corresponding hormonal triggers. A catamenial pattern has been reported most frequently with focal-onset seizures, but it can be seen in other types of seizures.

Progesterone Therapy

Cyclic progesterone therapy supplements progesterone during the luteal phase and withdraws it gradually premenstrually, as shown in **Box 1**. The NIH Progesterone Trial Treatment was a randomized, placebo-controlled, double-blind, clinical trial of progesterone in the treatment of intractable seizures in women with and without catamenial epilepsy.[11] Treatment consisted of baseline optimal AED therapy plus adjunctive natural progesterone lozenges or matching placebo. The findings of this trial showed that cyclic progesterone is comparable to placebo in the treatment of intractable seizures in women with focal-onset epilepsy.[11] A prespecified secondary analysis, however, identified a subset of women with perimenstrual seizure exacerbation (C1) of greater than or equal to 3-fold who were responsive to progesterone treatment. The detection of a greater than or equal to 3-fold level of perimenstrual seizure exacerbation might suggest a favorable response to treatment with adjunctive cyclic progesterone.[10] Cyclic progesterone supplement may have greater efficacy where progesterone withdrawal (C1) is implicated.[10] Potential adverse effects of natural progesterone lozenges include sedation, depression, asthenia, weight gain, irregular vaginal bleeding, and constipation.[10]

Table 1			
Patterns of catamenial epilepsy			
Catamenial Pattern	Menstrual Cycle Days	Menstrual Cycle Phase	Hormonal Changes
C1	−3 to 3	Perimenstrually	↓Progesterone
C2	10 to −13	Periovulatory	↑Estrogen
C3	10 to 3	Inadequate luteal phase	↑Estrogen/progesterone ratio

> **Box 1**
> **Cyclic progesterone treatment**
>
> Natural progesterone lozenges (200 mg)
>
> Instructions (day 1 = 1st day of menses)
>   1 Lozenge TID, days 14 to 25
>   ½ Lozenge TID, days 26 to 27
>   ¼ Lozenge TID, day 28
>   Stop day 29

Medroxyprogesterone acetate, a synthetic progesterone compound administered via intramuscular injection, may lower seizure frequency when it is given in sufficient dosage to induce amenorrhea.[12] Although it and other synthetic progestins are not metabolized to the inhibitory neurosteroid allopregnanolone, the benefit is thought to be due to eliminating the fluctuation of endogenous sex steroid hormones. In 1 open-label study of 14 women with refractory focal-onset seizures and normal ovulatory cycles, medroxyprogesterone administration in doses large enough to induce amenorrhea resulted in a 39% seizure reduction.[12] Side effects include those encountered with natural progesterone as well as hot flashes and a delay in return of regular ovulatory cycles and fertility. Long-term hypoestrogenic effects on cardiovascular status, bone density, and emotional health need to be considered with chronic use. Oral synthetic progestins administered cyclically or continuously have not proved effective therapy for seizures.[12,13]

Other Treatments

Acetazolamide has been used to treat catamenial epilepsy, but it has not been assessed in randomized trials. Effectiveness at doses of 250 mg to 500 mg daily administered for 3 to 7 days, starting approximately 3 days before menses, has been reported.[14] Clobazam has been formally studied for the treatment of catamenial epilepsy. In a double-blind, placebo-controlled, crossover study, clobazam was associated with better control than placebo. Complete control was seen in most patients during a 10-day treatment phase beginning 7 to 2 days before the menstrual flow adjusted for each patient so that treatment would begin 2 to 4 days before the time during which the exacerbation of epilepsy usually occurred.[15] A temporary increase in the dose of a patient's usual AEDs at specific times during the menstrual cycle is another reasonable, empirical approach, although phenytoin should not be increased due to the risk of toxic effects associated with its nonlinear kinetics.[2]

REPRODUCTIVE AND SEXUAL DYSFUNCTION

Increased rates of infertility have been reported in some studies of women with epilepsy, but other studies have reported normal fertility. Some of the postulated mechanisms for reduced fertility are related to the effect of epilepsy on reproductive hormones. Regions of the limbic cortex, in particular the amygdala, have reciprocal connections with the hypothalamus and can modulate the hypothalamic-pituitary-ovarian axis.[2] GnRH is produced by a population of cells in the preoptic area of the hypothalamus, which is vulnerable to injury by seizures. Dysfunction of GnRH cells is followed by the abnormal release of FSH and LH.[2] This phenomenon is known as hypogonadotropic hypogonadism.

EFFECT OF ANTIEPILEPTIC DRUGS ON REPRODUCTIVE HORMONES

Enzyme-inducing AEDs alter hepatic metabolism and decrease concentrations of reproductive hormones. They also induce production of sex hormone–binding globulin, which reduces concentrations of free reproductive hormones in serum.[2] Lofgren and colleagues[16] reported low total testosterone concentrations and free androgen indices in men with epilepsy taking carbamazepine or oxcarbazepine. Low total testosterone and free androgen levels may result in decreased sex drive.

Some AEDs directly alter hormonal production. For example, valproate has been reported to induce androgen synthesis in the ovaries.[2,17] This drug is associated with increased testosterone concentrations, anovulation, and polycystic ovarian syndrome.

EFFECT OF REPRODUCTIVE HORMONES ON ANTIEPILEPTIC DRUGS

On the other hand, levels of AEDs may fluctuate during the menstrual cycle due to hormonal effects. High levels of circulating estrogen in the luteal phase could theoretically induce hepatic isoenzymes used for AED metabolism, especially for glucuronidation, and thereby lower the level of circulating AED premenstrually; 1 study suggested minor changes in lamotrigine and valproate levels but findings were not significant.[18]

CONTRACEPTION

Pharmacokinetics of AEDs and hormonal contraceptives can interact bidirectionally, potentially increasing the elimination rate of either drug. The most widely used contraceptives are combined oral contraceptive (COC) formulations containing an estrogen and a progestin compound, but other hormonal contraceptives include progestin-only pills (POPs), patches, and vaginal rings, which work by secretion of an estrogen and progestin into the blood circulation, subcutaneous progestin implants, and intramuscular progestin injections. AEDs with a potential for hepatic enzyme induction—included in **Fig. 2**—may accelerate the hepatic metabolism of COCs and other hormonal contraceptives. The non–enzyme-inducing AEDs do not influence hormonal contraceptive metabolism and, therefore, can be administered without risk of contraceptive failure.

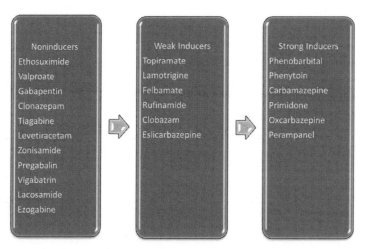

Fig. 2. Degree of induction of sex steroid hormones metabolism.

Combined OCs can increase the elimination of AEDs that are metabolized by glucuronidation. Among AEDs, this metabolic pathway has been studied most intensively for lamotrigine. The metabolism of lamotrigine is accelerated approximately 50% by cotreatment with COCs.[19] The clearance of valproic acid is also increased with COCs.[18] This information applies to other hormonal forms of birth control, including the vaginal ring and patch.

Only sparse data are available about possible interactions between AEDs and POPs. Enzyme-inducing AEDs increase the metabolism of progestins as well as estrogens; thus, POPs are not adequately efficacious when taken with enzyme-inducing AEDs. For women taking enzyme-inducing AEDs, an intrauterine device (IUD) is an excellent choice, and, given the safety and high contraceptive efficacy, an IUD is a favorable option for all women with epilepsy of reproductive age.[20] The levonorgestrel IUD prevents pregnancy by local hormonally mediated changes and is unlikely to be impacted by enzyme-inducing AEDs. Intramuscular medroxyprogesterone acetate is another long-acting reversible contraceptive that is likely adequate with coadministration of enzyme-inducing AEDs, because the concentration of progestin is high enough that efficacy is maintained but is often not considered a first-line option due to its side effects.

PREGNANCY

Epilepsy is the most common neurologic disorder that requires continuous treatment during pregnancy, and AEDs are one of the most frequent teratogen exposures.[20] Approximately 1.5 million women with epilepsy are of childbearing age in the United States, and 3 to 5 births per 1000 will be to women with epilepsy.[21] In a large observational study of women with epilepsy, approximately 52% of patients had seizures during pregnancy.[22] AED treatment during pregnancy is a balancing act between teratogenic risks to the fetus and maintaining maternal seizure control.

Risk of Congenital Malformations with Antiepileptic Drug Use

Major congenital malformations (MCMs) are defined as birth defects that are life threatening, have a major impact on the person, and/or require surgical treatment. The reported MCM rates in the general population vary between 1.6% and 3.2%, and women with epilepsy not receiving AEDs show similar rates.[20] The average MCM rates among all AED exposures vary between 3.1% and 9%, approximately 2-fold to 3-fold higher than in the general population.[23]

Minor anomalies are defined as structural deviations from the norm that do not constitute a health threat. Minor anomalies affect 6% to 20% of infants born to women with epilepsy, approximately 2.5-fold the rate of the general population.[20] Some examples of minor anomalies are ocular hypterteleroism, micrognathia, syndactyly, and polydactyly.

Antiepileptic Drug Monotherapies

A high risk of MCMs with first-trimester valproate exposure has been found in several large pregnancy registries.[24–27] The relative risk of MCMs with first-trimester exposure to valproate is approximately 3-fold, and the absolute risk is 6% to 9%.[28] For individual MCMs, many are elevated for valproate and include spina bifida. A publication from the North American AED Pregnancy Registry (NAAPR) revealed that phenobarbital also has a significantly increased risk of MCMs, most often cardiac defects.[29] If possible, both valproate and phenobarbital should be avoided in women of childbearing potential. There is a dose-associated risk for valproate and, in women who need these AEDs for seizure control and whose seizures have failed to respond adequately to all other AEDs, the smallest dose possible should be used.

In a 2010 study using the European Surveillance of Congenital Anomalies antiepileptic study database and incorporating other published reports, the findings suggested an association between spina bifida and in utero carbamazepine exposure compared with no exposure (odds ratio 2.6; 95% CI, 1.2–5.3).[30] The risk with carbamazepine, however, was approximately 80% less than with valproate.

Another important recent finding is the association of facial clefts with in utero topiramate exposure. The rate of oral clefts with first-trimester exposure to topiramate was 1.4% in the NAAPR, which is an approximately 10-fold increase compared with the control population prevalence of 0.11%.[29] As a point of comparison, in this report, oral cleft prevalence was 0.5% with lamotrigine, carbamazepine, and phenytoin; 1.2% with valproate; and 4% with phenobarbital.[29] This increased risk was also found in other large birth defect registries in the United States and in the UK Epilepsy and Pregnancy Register.[28,31] Emerging findings also suggest an association between topiramate use and hypospadias in exposed offspring.[32]

In the same NAAPR publication, the risk of MCMs with first-trimester exposures to lamotrigine, levetiracetam, carbamazepine, or phenytoin was between 2% and 2.5% for each individual drug.[29] Although there were not enough exposures to oxcarbazepine, gabapentin, or zonisamide in this study to determine precise estimates, the upper limits of the 95% CIs were low.[28] **Table 2** shows the risk of MCMs with exposure to each specific AED monotherapy during the first trimester, and **Table 3** summarizes the relative risk of MCMs with exposure to a specific AED monotherapy during the first trimester compared with unexposed and lamotrigine groups.[29]

Polytherapy

MCM rates have been reported higher for AED polytherapy compared with monotherapy regimens,[33] leading to the American Academy of Neurology and American Epilepsy Society (AAN-AES) Practice Parameter recommendation that AED monotherapy is preferred to polytherapy during pregnancy, and monotherapy should

Table 2 Risk of major congenital malformations with exposure to a specific antiepileptic drug monotherapy during the first trimester as reported by the North American AED Pregnancy Registry, 1997–2011	
Antiepileptic Drug Monotherapy	Major Congenital Malformations, No. (%) and 95% CI
Unexposed (n = 442)	5 (1.1), 0.37–2.6
Lamotrigine (n = l562)	31 (2.0), 1.4–2.8
Carbamazepine (n = l033)	31 (3.0), 2.1–4.2
Phenytoin (n = 416)	12 (2.9), 1.5–5.0
Levetiracetam (n = 450)	11 (2.4), 1.2–4.3
Topiramate (n = 359)	15 (4.2), 2.4–6.8
Valproate (n = 323)	30 (9.3), 6.4–13.0
Phenobarbital (n = 199)	11 (5.5), 2.8–9.7
Oxcarbazepine (n = 182)	4 (2.2), 0.6–5.5
Gabapentin (n = 145)	1 (0.7), 0.02–3.8
Zonisamide (n = 90)	0 (0), 0.0–3.3
Clonazepam (n = 64)	2 (3.1), 0.4–10.8

Table 3
Relative risk of major congenital malformations with exposure to a specific antiepileptic drug monotherapy during the first trimester, compared with unexposed and lamotrigine groups, as reported by the North American AED Pregnancy Registry, 1997–2011

Antiepileptic Drug Monotherapy	Unexposed Reference Relative Risk, 95% CI	Exposed Reference Relative Risk, 95% CI
Lamotrigine (n = I562)	1.8, 0.7–4.6	Reference
Carbamazepine (n = 1033)	2.7, 1.0–7.0	1.5, 0.9–2.5
Phenytoin (n = 416)	2.6, 0.9–7.4	1.5, 0.7–2.9
Levetiracetam (n = 450)	2.2, 0.8–6.4	1.2, 0.6–2.5
Topiramate (n = 359)	3.8, 1.4–1.06	2.2, 1.2–4.0
Valproate (n = 323)	9.0, 3.4–23.3	5.1, 3.0–8.5
Phenobarbital (n = 199)	5.1, 1.8–14.9	2.9, 1.4–5.8
Oxcarbazepine (n = 182)	2.0, 0.5–7.4	1.1, 0.4–3.1
Gabapentin (n = 145)	0.6, 0.07–5.2	0.3, 0.05–2.5
Zonisamide (n = 90)	N/A	N/A
Clonazepam (n = 64)	2.8, 0.5–14.8	1.6, 0.4–6.8

Unexposed Reference = Relative risk of major congenital malformations with exposure to each specific antiepileptic drug monotherapy during the first trimester, compared with unexposed subjects or subjects not exposed to antiepileptic drug(s).

Exposed reference = Relative risk of major congenital malformations with exposure to each specific antiepileptic drug monotherapy during the first trimester, compared with subjects exposed to lamotrigine.

Abbreviation: N/A, not available, relative risk not available due to insufficient data.

be achieved during the preconception phase.[33] Since this Practice Parameter, however, new data suggest that this could be an oversimplification. Data from the NAAPR suggest that not all AED polytherapy combinations are the same. Both lamotrigine and carbamazepine had relatively low MCM rates in polytherapy regimens that did not contain valproate. The MCM rate for lamotrigine was 2.9% with any AED other than valproate but 9.1% for lamotrigine combined with valproate. Similarly, the MCM rate for carbamazepine was 2.5% with any AED other than valproate, but 15.4% for carbamazepine combined with valproate.

Cognitive and Behavioral Teratogenesis of Antiepileptic Drugs

Studies investigating cognitive outcomes in children of women with epilepsy suggest an increased risk of mental impairment.[33] Verbal scores on neuropsychometric measures may be selectively more involved.[34] Although a variety of factors contribute to the cognitive problems of children of women with epilepsy, AEDs seem to play a major role. AED-induced functional and anatomic defects may involve different mechanisms because anatomic risks are related to first-trimester exposure, and functional deficits may be related primarily to third-trimester exposure or at least exposure throughout the entire pregnancy. AEDs that are known to induce apoptosis, such as valproate, seem to affect children's neurodevelopment in a more severe fashion.[35,36] The results of the Neurodevelopmental Effects of Antiepileptic Drugs (NEAD) study revealed that fetal valproate exposure has dose-dependent associations with reduced cognitive abilities across a range of domains, including low IQ, and these seem to persist at least until the age of 6.[37] Some studies have shown neurodevelopmental deficiencies, including low verbal intelligence, associated with the use of phenobarbital and possibly phenytoin.[38–42] So far, most of the investigations available suggest that fetal exposures to lamotrigine or levetiracetam are safer with regard to cognition compared with other AEDs.[37,43,44] Studies on carbamazepine exposure show consistent results that support normal neurodevelopment, leading to an AAN-AES practice parameter that concludes this AED probably does not increase poor cognitive outcome compared with unexposed controls.[32,33,36] Overall, children exposed to polytherapy prenatally seem to have worse cognitive and behavioral outcomes than children exposed to monotherapy.[45–47] There is an increased risk of neurodevelopmental deficits when polytherapy involves the use of valproate versus other agents.[48] In addition, the Liverpool and Manchester Neurodevelopment Group reported findings suggesting that valproate may be associated with autism spectrum disorder. In their small sample, 6.3% of the children exposed to valproate monotherapy had clinically diagnosed autism spectrum disorder.[49] This is 7-fold higher than the control group and more than 10-fold higher than the reported incidence in the general population. Additional evidence comes from a study by Christensen and colleagues,[50] in which the absolute risk of autism spectrum disorder among 432 children exposed to valproate was 4.15% (95% CI, 2.20–7.81), and the absolute risk of childhood autism was 2.95% (95% CI, 1.42–6.11).

Other Birth Outcomes

Chen and colleagues[51] reported that seizures in women with epilepsy during pregnancy were associated with a 1.5-fold increase for preterm delivery or infants being small for gestational age. A secondary analysis of the neonatal outcomes from the NEAD cohort reported that adverse neonatal outcome risks may differ between the AEDs; the odds ratio for infants being born small for gestational age was higher for the valproate and carbamazepine groups, and reduced 1-minute Apgar scores occurred more frequently in the phenytoin and valproate groups.[52] More recently, findings from the NAAPR suggested an association between in utero exposure to zonisamide and topiramate and a decrease in mean birth weight and length.[53] Prenatal exposure to topiramate or zonisamide was associated with mean lower birth weights of 221 g and 202 g, respectively, and a mean lesser neonatal length of 1 cm compared with lamotrigine exposure ($P<.1$). The prevalence of small for gestational age was 6.8% for lamotrigine, 17.9% for topiramate (RR 2.4; 95% CI, 1.8–3.3), and 12.2% for zonisamide (RR 1.6; 95% CI 0.9%–2.8%). Similar results were found when a group of 457 unexposed neonates was used as a reference.

Folic Acid Use

Folic acid supplementation in women in the general population during pregnancy has been associated with a risk reduction in the occurrence of congenital malformations, including neural tube defects.[54] In addition, the NEAD study showed higher mean IQs in the children of mothers who took periconceptional folic acid supplementation in addition to folic acid later during pregnancy.[37] Although in the past some organizations advocated that women on treatment with AEDs associated with a higher risk of neural tube defects took a folic acid dose of 4 mg per day, the effectiveness of this dose versus lower doses in the absence of a family history of neural tube defects has not been established.

Antiepileptic Drug Metabolism and Management During Pregnancy

Many of the AEDs undergo enhanced clearance during pregnancy and the serum concentrations need to be monitored. Per the 2009 AAN-AES Practice Parameter, it seems reasonable to individualize this monitoring for each patient with the aim of maintaining a level near the preconceptional level, presumably at which the women with epilepsy were doing well with seizure control.[20] A proposed approach is to check AED serum levels monthly and adjust the dose to compensate for significant declines. Studies have indicated that a decrease in the concentration to 65% or less of an individual's target concentration is associated with increased risk of seizure worsening.[55,56] Postpartum, the AED should be gradually tapered to the preconception dose to avoid supratherapeutic levels and toxicity. Different approaches may be used to accomplish this taper adapted to the particular AED. The postpartum pharmacokinetic changes and clinical consequences are best documented for lamotrigine, and the adjustment in dose should begin within 3 days postpartum with return to preconception dose or slightly higher to accommodate sleep-deprivation effects within 10 to 21 days postpartum.[56] Postpartum pharmacokinetic changes with AEDs that are metabolized primarily by the cytochrome p450 system likely occur more gradually.[57]

A range of physiologic changes during gestation may alter the pharmacokinetics of AEDs.[58] Increased volume of distribution may lead to reduced AED serum concentrations. Increased renal blood flow and glomerular filtration rate may reduce the serum concentrations of AEDs predominantly eliminated via the kidneys. Reduced serum albumin concentrations may affect AED protein binding and plasma clearance. Increased estrogen levels lead to accelerated drug glucuronidation.[59] In addition, the activity of some cytochrome P450 enzymes is increased.[60] Lamotrigine, one of the most commonly used AEDs during pregnancy, is extensively metabolized by glucuronidation. Its clearance in the last trimester of pregnancy increases to an average of double compared with baseline, with a reduction in the dose-normalized serum concentration by 40% to 60%.[61–65] A more in-depth pharmacokinetic modeling study of lamotrigine demonstrated, however, that 77% of women had a greater than 3-fold increase in clearance during pregnancy whereas 23% had only a minimal increase, and the investigators postulated that the subpopulations may be due to pharmacogenetic differences.[56] The interindividual variability is another argument for the use of therapeutic drug monitoring during pregnancy.

Oxcarbazepine is metabolized to the pharmacologically active monohydroxycarbazepine, which is eliminated as a glucoronide. In 2 small studies, the serum concentrations of monohydroxycarbazepine were at least 36% lower during pregnancy compared with prepregnancy or postpregnancy values.[66,67] One-third of an oral dose of levetiracetam is metabolized in blood by hydrolysis and two-thirds are usually found unchanged in the urine. The clearance of levetiracetam increases significantly during pregnancy. Case series have demonstrated reduced serum concentration as low as 50% of baseline.[68,69]

BREASTFEEDING

Estimates of AED exposure from breast milk suggest that it is low for many AEDs.[70] Data on AED serum levels in the breastfeeding child are sparse, however, except for lamotrigine. In a study of 30 mother-child pairs, infant plasma concentrations were 18.3% of maternal plasma concentrations.[71] No adverse effects of AED exposure via breastmilk were observed at age 6 in the NEAD study. In addition, breastfed children in this study exhibited a higher IQ and enhanced verbal abilities.[72] As a general rule, breastfeeding is recommended to mothers with epilepsy based on the known positive effects of breastfeeding and lack of scientific evidence to support the theoretic risks.

MENOPAUSE

Increased rates of premature menopause characterized by amenorrhea and ovarian failure have been reported in women with focal-onset epilepsy of temporal lobe origin.[73] In a 1986 survey of women with epilepsy by Herzog and colleagues,[73] 2 of 50 women had an onset of menopause before age 40, which is much higher than the expected rate of less than 1% in the general population. In a study by Harden and colleagues[74] (2003), the median age of menopause was 47 years among women with epilepsy compared with 51.4 years in the background population, and seizure frequency or lifetime number of seizures was associated with the timing of cessation of reproductive cycling.[74] Hormone replacement therapy is associated with a dose-related increase in seizure frequency in postmenopausal women with epilepsy.[75]

SUMMARY

Optimal treatment of women with epilepsy requires an understanding of the complex interactions of sex steroid hormones with epilepsy and AEDs, and the potential risks of AEDs during pregnancy. Informed treatment recommendations provide improved seizure control with fewer adverse effects for women with epilepsy and their offspring.

REFERENCES

1. Gu Q, Moss RL. 17 beta-Estradiol potentiates kainate-induced currents via activation of the cAMP cascade. J Neurosci 1996;16(11):3620–9.
2. Harden CL, Pennell PB. Neuroendocrine considerations in the treatment of men and women with epilepsy. Lancet Neurol 2013;12(1):72–83.
3. Weiland NG. Estradiol selectively regulates agonist binding sites on the N-methyl-D-aspartate receptor complex in the CA1 region of the hippocampus. Endocrinology 1992;131(2):662–8.
4. Reddy DS, Rogawski MA. Neurosteroids - endogenous regulators of seizure susceptibility and role in the treatment of epilepsy. In: Noebels JL, Avoli M, Rogawski MA, et al, editors. Jasper's basic mechanisms of the epilepsies. 4th edition. New York: Oxford University Press; 2012. p. 984–97.
5. Majewska MD, Harrison NL, Schwartz RD, et al. Steroid hormone metabolites are barbiturate-like modulators of the GABA receptor. Science 1986;232(4753): 1004–7.
6. Pennell PB. Hormonal aspects of epilepsy. Neurol Clin 2009;27(4):941–65.
7. Herzog AG, Klein P, Ransil BJ. Three patterns of catamenial epilepsy. Epilepsia 1997;38(10):1082–8.
8. Jones GS. Luteal phase defect: a review of pathophysiology. Curr Opin Obstet Gynecol 1991;3(5):641–8.
9. Herzog AG. Catamenial epilepsy: definition, prevalence pathophysiology and treatment. Seizure 2008;17(2):151–9.
10. Herzog AG. Catamenial epilepsy: update on prevalence, pathophysiology and treatment from the findings of the NIH progesterone treatment trial. Seizure 2015;28:18–25.
11. Herzog AG, Fowler KM, Smithson SD, et al. Progesterone vs placebo therapy for women with epilepsy: a randomized clinical trial. Neurology 2012;78(24): 1959–66.
12. Mattson RH, Cramer JA, Caldwell BV, et al. Treatment of seizures with medroxy-progesterone acetate: preliminary report. Neurology 1984;34(9):1255–8.
13. Dana-Haeri J, Richens A. Effect of norethisterone on seizures associated with menstruation. Epilepsia 1983;24(3):377–81.
14. Ansell B, Clarke E. Acetazolamide in treatment of epilepsy. Br Med J 1956; 1(4968):650–4.

15. Feely M, Calvert R, Gibson J. Clobazam in catamenial epilepsy. A model for evaluating anticonvulsants. Lancet 1982;2(8289):71–3.

16. Lofgren E, Tapanainen JS, Koivunen R, et al. Effects of carbamazepine and oxcarbazepine on the reproductive endocrine function in women with epilepsy. Epilepsia 2006;47(9):1441–6.

17. Nelson-DeGrave VL, Wickenheisser JK, Cockrell JE, et al. Valproate potentiates androgen biosynthesis in human ovarian theca cells. Endocrinology 2004; 145(2):799–808.

18. Herzog AG, Blum AS, Farina EL, et al. Valproate and lamotrigine level variation with menstrual cycle phase and oral contraceptive use. Neurology 2009;72(10): 911–4.

19. Christensen J, Petrenaite V, Atterman J, et al. Oral contraceptives induce lamotrigine metabolism: evidence from a double-blind, placebo-controlled trial. Epilepsia 2007;48(3):484–9.

20. Pennell PB. Pregnancy, epilepsy, and women's issues. Continuum (Minneap Minn) 2013;19(3 Epilepsy):697–714.

21. Harden CL, Pennell PB, Koppel BS, et al. Practice parameter update: management issues for women with epilepsy–focus on pregnancy (an evidence-based review): vitamin K, folic acid, blood levels, and breastfeeding: report of the Quality Standards Subcommittee and Therapeutics and Technology Assessment Subcommittee of the American Academy of Neurology and American Epilepsy Society. Neurology 2009;73(2):142–9.

22. Thomas SV, Syam U, Devi JS. Predictors of seizures during pregnancy in women with epilepsy. Epilepsia 2012;53(5):e85–8.

23. Pennell PB. Antiepileptic drugs during pregnancy: what is known and which AEDs seem to be safest? Epilepsia 2008;49(Suppl 9):43–55.

24. Morrow J, Russell A, Guthrie E, et al. Malformation risks of antiepileptic drugs in pregnancy: a prospective study from the UK Epilepsy and Pregnancy Register. J Neurol Neurosurg Psychiatry 2006;77(2):193–8.

25. Wide K, Winbladh B, Kallen B. Major malformations in infants exposed to antiepileptic drugs in utero, with emphasis on carbamazepine and valproic acid: a nation-wide, population-based register study. Acta Paediatr 2004;93(2):174–6.

26. Artama M, Auvinen A, Raudaskoski T, et al. Antiepileptic drug use of women with epilepsy and congenital malformations in offspring. Neurology 2005;64(11): 1874–8.

27. Campbell E, Kennedy F, Russell A, et al. Malformation risks of antiepileptic drug monotherapies in pregnancy: updated results from the UK and Ireland Epilepsy and Pregnancy Registers. J Neurol Neurosurg Psychiatry 2014; 85(9):1029–34.

28. Harden CL. Pregnancy and epilepsy. Continuum (Minneap Minn) 2014;20(1 Neurology of Pregnancy):60–79.

29. Hernandez-Diaz S, Smith CR, Shen A, et al. Comparative safety of antiepileptic drugs during pregnancy. Neurology 2012;78(21):1692–9.

30. Jentink J, Dolk H, Loane MA, et al. Intrauterine exposure to carbamazepine and specific congenital malformations: systematic review and case-control study. BMJ 2010;341:c6581.

31. Margulis AV, Mitchell AA, Gilboa SM, et al. Use of topiramate in pregnancy and risk of oral clefts. Am J Obstet Gynecol 2012;207(5):405.e1–7.

32. Vajda FJ, O'Brien TJ, Graham J, et al. Associations between particular types of fetal malformation and antiepileptic drug exposure in utero. Acta Neurol Scand 2013;128(4):228–34.

33. Harden CL, Meador KJ, Pennell PB, et al. Management issues for women with epilepsy-focus on pregnancy (an evidence-based review): II. Teratogenesis and perinatal outcomes: report of the quality standards subcommittee and therapeutics and technology subcommittee of the American Academy of Neurology and the American Epilepsy Society. Epilepsia 2009;50(5):1237–46.
34. Meador KJ, Baker GA, Browning N, et al. Foetal antiepileptic drug exposure and verbal versus non-verbal abilities at three years of age. Brain 2011;134(Pt 2): 396–404.
35. Bittigau P, Sifringer M, Genz K, et al. Antiepileptic drugs and apoptotic neurodegeneration in the developing brain. Proc Natl Acad Sci U S A 2002;99(23): 15089–94.
36. Bittigau P, Sifringer M, Ikonomidou C. Antiepileptic drugs and apoptosis in the developing brain. Ann N Y Acad Sci 2003;993:103–14 [discussion: 123–4].
37. Meador KJ, Baker GA, Browning N, et al. Fetal antiepileptic drug exposure and cognitive outcomes at age 6 years (NEAD study): a prospective observational study. Lancet Neurol 2013;12(3):244–52.
38. Farwell JR, Lee YJ, Hirtz DG, et al. Phenobarbital for febrile seizures–effects on intelligence and on seizure recurrence. N Engl J Med 1990;322(6):364–9.
39. Reinisch JM, Sanders SA, Mortensen EL, et al. In utero exposure to phenobarbital and intelligence deficits in adult men. JAMA 1995;274(19):1518–25.
40. Sulzbacher S, Farwell JR, Temkin N, et al. Late cognitive effects of early treatment with phenobarbital. Clin Pediatr (Phila) 1999;38(7):387–94.
41. Vanoverloop D, Schnell RR, Harvey EA, et al. The effects of prenatal exposure to phenytoin and other anticonvulsants on intellectual function at 4 to 8 years of age. Neurotoxicol Teratol 1992;14(5):329–35.
42. Scolnik D, Nulman I, Rovet J, et al. Neurodevelopment of children exposed in utero to phenytoin and carbamazepine monotherapy. JAMA 1994;271(10): 767–70.
43. Shallcross R, Bromley RL, Cheyne CP, et al. In utero exposure to levetiracetam vs valproate: development and language at 3 years of age. Neurology 2014;82(3): 213–21.
44. Shallcross R, Bromley RL, Irwin B, et al. Child development following in utero exposure: levetiracetam vs sodium valproate. Neurology 2011;76(4):383–9.
45. Forsberg L, Wide K, Kallen B. School performance at age 16 in children exposed to antiepileptic drugs in utero–a population-based study. Epilepsia 2011;52(2): 364–9.
46. Koch S, Titze K, Zimmermann RB, et al. Long-term neuropsychological consequences of maternal epilepsy and anticonvulsant treatment during pregnancy for school-age children and adolescents. Epilepsia 1999;40(9):1237–43.
47. Losche G, Steinhausen HC, Koch S, et al. The psychological development of children of epileptic parents. II. The differential impact of intrauterine exposure to anticonvulsant drugs and further influential factors. Acta Paediatr 1994;83(9):961–6.
48. Nadebaum C, Anderson V, Vajda F, et al. The Australian brain and cognition and antiepileptic drugs study: IQ in school-aged children exposed to sodium valproate and polytherapy. J Int Neuropsychol Soc 2011;17(1):133–42.
49. Bromley RL, Mawer GE, Briggs M, et al. The prevalence of neurodevelopmental disorders in children prenatally exposed to antiepileptic drugs. J Neurol Neurosurg Psychiatry 2013;84(6):637–43.
50. Christensen J, Gronborg TK, Sorensen MJ, et al. Prenatal valproate exposure and risk of autism spectrum disorders and childhood autism. JAMA 2013;309(16): 1696–703.

51. Chen YH, Chiou HY, Lin HC, et al. Affect of seizures during gestation on pregnancy outcomes in women with epilepsy. Arch Neurol 2009;66(8):979–84.

52. Pennell PB, Klein AM, Browning N, et al. Differential effects of antiepileptic drugs on neonatal outcomes. Epilepsy Behav 2012;24(4):449–56.

53. Hernandez-Diaz S, Mittendorf R, Smith CR, et al. Association between topiramate and zonisamide use during pregnancy and low birth weight. Obstet Gynecol 2014;123(1):21–8.

54. Czeizel AE. Periconceptional folic acid and multivitamin supplementation for the prevention of neural tube defects and other congenital abnormalities. Birth Defects Res A Clin Mol Teratol 2009;85(4):260–8.

55. Reisinger TL, Newman M, Loring DW, et al. Antiepileptic drug clearance and seizure frequency during pregnancy in women with epilepsy. Epilepsy Behav 2013;29(1):13–8.

56. Polepally AR, Pennell PB, Brundage RC, et al. Model-based lamotrigine clearance changes during pregnancy: clinical implication. Ann Clin Transl Neurol 2014;1(2):99–106.

57. Pennell PB, Hovinga CA. Antiepileptic drug therapy in pregnancy I: gestation-induced effects on AED pharmacokinetics. Int Rev Neurobiol 2008;83:227–40.

58. Brodtkorb E, Reimers A. Seizure control and pharmacokinetics of antiepileptic drugs in pregnant women with epilepsy. Seizure 2008;17(2):160–5.

59. Reimers A, Brodtkorb E. Second-generation antiepileptic drugs and pregnancy: a guide for clinicians. Expert Rev Neurother 2012;12(6):707–17.

60. Anderson GD. Pregnancy-induced changes in pharmacokinetics: a mechanistic-based approach. Clin Pharmacokinet 2005;44(10):989–1008.

61. de Haan GJ, Edelbroek P, Segers J, et al. Gestation-induced changes in lamotrigine pharmacokinetics: a monotherapy study. Neurology 2004;63(3):571–3.

62. Ohman I, Vitols S, Tomson T. Lamotrigine in pregnancy: pharmacokinetics during delivery, in the neonate, and during lactation. Epilepsia 2000;41(6):709–13.

63. Pennell PB, Newport DJ, Stowe ZN, et al. The impact of pregnancy and childbirth on the metabolism of lamotrigine. Neurology 2004;62(2):292–5.

64. Petrenaite V, Sabers A, Hansen-Schwartz J. Individual changes in lamotrigine plasma concentrations during pregnancy. Epilepsy Res 2005;65(3):185–8.

65. Tran TA, Leppik IE, Blesi K, et al. Lamotrigine clearance during pregnancy. Neurology 2002;59(2):251–5.

66. Mazzucchelli I, Onat FY, Ozkara C, et al. Changes in the disposition of oxcarbazepine and its metabolites during pregnancy and the puerperium. Epilepsia 2006;47(3):504–9.

67. Christensen J, Sabers A, Sidenius P. Oxcarbazepine concentrations during pregnancy: a retrospective study in patients with epilepsy. Neurology 2006;67(8):1497–9.

68. Tomson T, Palm R, Kallen K, et al. Pharmacokinetics of levetiracetam during pregnancy, delivery, in the neonatal period, and lactation. Epilepsia 2007;48(6):1111–6.

69. Westin AA, Reimers A, Helde G, et al. Serum concentration/dose ratio of levetiracetam before, during and after pregnancy. Seizure 2008;17(2):192–8.

70. Hovinga CA, Pennell PB. Antiepileptic drug therapy in pregnancy II: fetal and neonatal exposure. Int Rev Neurobiol 2008;83:241–58.

71. Newport DJ, Pennell PB, Calamaras MR, et al. Lamotrigine in breast milk and nursing infants: determination of exposure. Pediatrics 2008;122(1):e223–31.

72. Meador KJ, Baker GA, Browning N, et al. Breastfeeding in children of women taking antiepileptic drugs: cognitive outcomes at age 6 years. JAMA Pediatr 2014;168(8):729–36.

73. Herzog AG, Seibel MM, Schomer DL, et al. Reproductive endocrine disorders in women with partial seizures of temporal lobe origin. Arch Neurol 1986;43(4): 341–6.
74. Harden CL, Koppel BS, Herzog AG, et al. Seizure frequency is associated with age at menopause in women with epilepsy. Neurology 2003;61(4):451–5.
75. Harden CL, Herzog AG, Nikolov BG, et al. Hormone replacement therapy in women with epilepsy: a randomized, double-blind, placebo-controlled study. Epilepsia 2006;47(9):1447–51.

Counseling Epilepsy Patients on Driving and Employment

Allan Krumholz, MD*, Jennifer L. Hopp, MD, Ana M. Sanchez, MD

KEYWORDS

- Driving • Employment • Automobile • Disability • Work • Accidents • Licensure
- Unemployment

KEY POINTS

- Driving and employment are among their major concerns for people with epilepsy. Physicians are involved as health care providers, as advisors to people with epilepsy, and as consultants to employers and regulatory authorities.
- For people with seizures, the seizure-free interval is the key standard in determining licensure to drive, and generally varies from 3 to 12 months in the United States.
- Clinicians neither grant nor suspend driving privileges; this is the sole legal prerogative of the state. Physicians should counsel patients regarding the risks associated with driving and epilepsy and the applicable driving laws in their state.
- For people with seizures, most jobs, with reasonable accommodation by employers, are suitable. Categorical or blanket prohibitions to employment for seizures are generally not legal in the United States.
- Federal protections through the Americans with Disabilities Act confer civil rights protection by law on people with disabilities such as epilepsy and have opened more employment opportunities for people with epilepsy.

INTRODUCTION

Epilepsy is more than just a medical condition; it is also a serious social disorder. Seizures may limit an individual's productive participation in society. Such epilepsy-related social problems are emphasized in the recent comprehensive report from the Institute on Medicine entitled, *Epilepsy Across the Spectrum: Promoting Health and Understanding*.[1] Indeed, social and culture challenges for people with epilepsy

Disclosure Statement: The authors have nothing to disclose.

Department of Neurology, University of Maryland School of Medicine, Maryland Epilepsy Center, University of Maryland Medical Center, 22 South Greene Street, S12C09, Baltimore, MD 21201, USA

* Corresponding author.

E-mail address: akrumholz@som.umaryland.edu

Neurol Clin 34 (2016) 427–442

http://dx.doi.org/10.1016/j.ncl.2015.11.005

neurologic.theclinics.com

are not new. In ancient times, epilepsy and seizures were attributed to supernatural forces or demonic possession.[1,2] Nevertheless, today in many societies and cultures, persisting public misconceptions and stigmas about epilepsy and seizures limit opportunities. Without a doubt, people with epilepsy specifically identify social consequences of epilepsy and seizures, particularly problems with driving and employment, among their major concerns (**Fig. 1**).[3,4] Moreover, because epilepsy-associated social problems contribute to psychological comorbidities, including depression and anxiety, they also negatively quality of.[5] Physicians and other medical providers do not always recognize these problems. This article specifically addresses driving and employment for people with epilepsy to offer guidance for physicians and other medical providers regarding counseling of patients with seizure disorders and their families.

DRIVING

In the United States and many other countries, driving a car is critical to such key aspects of modern life as employment, socialization, and self-esteem.[6,7] Physicians are involved in the issues regarding driving and seizures in many ways: as health care providers, as advisors to people with epilepsy, and as consultants to regulatory authorities. Unfortunately, evidence indicates that patients with seizures are often not properly counseled by medical providers about rules and regulations regarding driving.[8,9]

Background

Despite the desire and necessity of many individuals with epilepsy to drive, seizures while driving pose risks for crashes that may result in property damage, injuries, and even deaths.[6,7] Factors such as duration of seizure freedom help predict the risk for crashes. Therefore, in the United States and most other countries, people with controlled epilepsy are permitted to drive, but only after review by regulatory authorities and with legal restrictions and monitoring.[6,7]

Epilepsy poses some driving risk, but that risk is limited, somewhat predictable, and relatively small compared with other causes of crashes, like alcohol.[6,7] For instance,

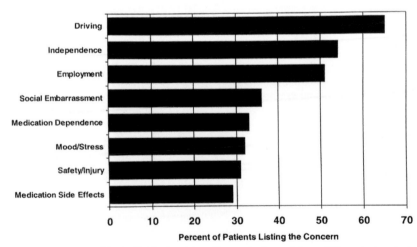

Fig. 1. Concerns noted by individuals with epilepsy. (*Adapted from* Gilliam F, Kuzniecky R, Faught E, et al. Patient-validated content of epilepsy-specific quality-of-life measurement. Epilepsia 1997;38:235.)

one study found that of all fatal driver crashes, only 0.2% are attributed to a seizure as compared with 30% for alcohol-related crashes.[10] In general, people with epilepsy have been shown to have a nearly 2-fold increased risk for crashing,[11–13] but that risk is for crashes of all causes rather than just seizure-related crashes. Indeed, only about 11% of all car crashes involving individuals with epilepsy are due to seizures,[12] with the great majority instead caused by the same thing that causes most crashes in the general population, which is simply driver error.[11,12,14] The risk of crashing for individuals with epilepsy based on large population-based studies is not substantially higher than for those with similar chronic medical conditions that are not as strictly regulated.[11–15] Evidence supports that having a seizure while driving is dangerous.[6,7] Therefore, patients with epilepsy or seizures should be advised that public policies regulating drivers with seizures, although limiting and far from ideal in many respects, are appropriate and necessary for the safety of the public and people with epilepsy.

Driving Standards, Regulations, and Practices

People with controlled seizures may be permitted to drive in every state in the United States, but people with uncontrolled seizures are restricted from licensure. The legal rules for determining control and administering restrictions are a complex mix of federal and state laws, regulations, and local practices that vary widely across the country.[16] The standards also change over time; updated information is available from local state authorities and on good informational sites, such as those of the Epilepsy Foundation (EF; https://www.epilepsy.com/driving-laws). In general, those rules aim to restrict driving by those with epilepsy who are at greatest risk for having seizures while driving. The key standard for determining that risk is the seizure-free interval, which is the duration of time a person with epilepsy has been seizure-free.[7,16] Essentially, the standard is that a person with a history of seizures or epilepsy may be licensed to drive if that individual has had no seizures for a time period adequate to demonstrate that a seizure recurrence while driving is of sufficiently low probability or risk. In the United States, the accepted time period for seizure freedom varies from about 3 months to 12 months, depending on individual state rules.[7,16] Some states give physicians great discretion, on an individualized basis, for recommending a specific period of seizure freedom or other requirements for licensing driving.[7,16]

Emphasis on the seizure-free interval as a key measure of safety to drive seems warranted and is widely supported.[7] One study showed that it is the strongest predictor for risk of seizure-related crashes in drivers with epilepsy.[17] Although it is generally accepted that the seizure-free interval is a key determinant for driving, the specific duration of a required seizure-free interval is the subject of considerable debate.[7,16] Scientific research on this is limited, but 6- to 12-month seizure-free intervals are reported to significantly reduce odds of crashing during a seizure compared with shorter intervals.[10] A 3-month seizure-free interval is proposed by the consensus statement from the American Academy of Neurology (AAN), American Epilepsy Society (AES), and the EF.[18]

Although the seizure-free interval is the key standard in determining licensure, other factors may also be considered.[6,7,16] For example, the consensus statement of the AAN, AES, and EF proposes several clinical mitigating factors to consider when determining whether a patient should be licensed to drive and how long a seizure-free interval to require. Favorable modifying factors that might lead to accepting a shorter seizure-free requirement or negating one completely include the following[18]:

- Seizures during medically directed changes in medication
- Focal seizures without alteration of awareness that do not interfere with consciousness or motor function

- Seizures that begin with consistent and prolonged auras
- Seizures related to acute toxic or metabolic states or illnesses that are not likely to recur

In contrast, proposed unfavorable modifiers that might lead to requiring a relatively longer seizure-free requirement and restricting driving include the following[18]:

- Noncompliance with medication or medical visits, or lack of credibility
- Recent history of active alcohol or drug abuse
- Structural brain disease
- Uncorrectable brain functional or metabolic disorder
- Frequent seizure recurrences after prior seizure-free intervals
- Prior crashes caused by seizures
- Previous bad driving record

Although these recommendations are based mainly on expert opinion, some scientific validation exists for this general approach. A comparison study confirmed that some of these factors, such as the seizure-free interval, reliable auras, and previous history of crashes, do correlate with the risk for seizure-related crashes.[16] However, another study questioned whether reliable auras are predictive of lower risk.[13]

Noncompliance with legal standards is a major limitation in effectively regulating drivers with medical conditions such as epilepsy.[5,7,17] Studies indicate that approximately half of all drivers do not report their epilepsy to regulators as required.[6,7,19–21] Noncompliance dilutes the public safety value of longer seizure-free intervals.[22] More permissive restrictions, such a short seizure-free interval, although potentially increasing an individual's risk of a crash, may actually reduce the cumulative risk by promoting better compliance with existing legal driving limitations in the general population (**Fig. 2**). In support of this, one study found that a 3-month seizure-free interval did not significantly increase the incidence of car crashes and deaths from seizures in the 3 years following implementation, as compared with a prior 1-year seizure-free requirement,[23] and another found no difference in driver fatalities in states with short compared with long seizure-free requirements.[10] Other studies and experts promote longer seizure-free intervals.[13,24–26]

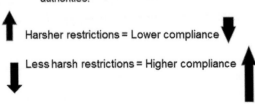

Noncompliance with Driving Regulations

- 40% to 60% of patients with epilepsy who drive do not report this condition to authorities.

Harsher restrictions = Lower compliance

Less harsh restrictions = Higher compliance

Fig. 2. Potential relations and interactions between the severity of driving restrictions with compliance with regulation.

Reporting Drivers with Epilepsy

All states except 6 in the United States do not require mandatory physician reporting of patients with seizures to the state motor vehicle administration. The states requiring mandatory reporting include California, Delaware, Nevada, New Jersey, Oregon, and Pennsylvania. Physician groups in the United States and elsewhere generally oppose such mandatory reporting, fearing that their patients will not be forthcoming about experiencing seizures, and thus be improperly treated. Indeed, patients with epilepsy frequently do not inform their physicians about their seizures, fearing loss of driving privileges and other social consequences.[6,16,18,27] One study comparing jurisdictions with and without such mandatory reporting provides some evidence that although mandatory physician reporting increases the percentage of patients with epilepsy known to regulators, it does not appear to reduce the risk of crashes or improve the public's safety.[28] However, other research considering several different medical disabilities including epilepsy notes that when physicians are incented to report drivers considered potentially unfit to drive to authorities, there is a subsequent decrease in subsequent trauma from road crashes, but that study also notes that this policy may also exacerbate mood disorders and compromise the doctor-patient relationship.[29]

Although mandatory physician reporting is not required in every state, self-reporting for individuals with seizures is mandated. The motor vehicle administrations of individual states administer this policy with specific rules varying among states. Patient noncompliance with required reporting is as a major limitation of this voluntary policy.[16–18,20,21,27–29]

Physicians in states that require mandatory reporting by physicians are obligated to do so. Apart from that, the counseling duties of physicians to their seizure patients regarding driving may be summarized as follows:

- Educate about the risks for driving with seizures.
- Inform about the legal rules and responsibilities for driving, including the duty to self-report.
- Explain that the decision as to when the patient can legally drive is not the medical providers but is that of the state's legal authorities, such as the Motor Vehicle Administration. Generally, medical providers make recommendations to that authority.
- Document such discussions in the patient's medical record.

In some instances, even in states without mandatory reporting, it may be appropriate for a clinician to report a patient driving with epilepsy to state authorities. As an example, a patient with uncontrolled seizures who crashes because of a seizure is at high risk for subsequent crashes. If such a patient refuses to self-report, providers should carefully consider reporting the patient to state authorities. In some states, physicians are legally protected for their recommendations and reports to the state; this is not true in every state, and medical providers should verify the updated legal standards in their own states. As recommended by expert opinion in the American Medical Association *Journal of Ethics*, "Physicians should be aware of their professional responsibilities and the legal requirements of the states in which they practice. When determining whether to report a patient's medical condition that may impair driving, physicians may have to weigh conflicting guidelines: a professional obligation to report and a legal requirement to maintain confidentiality, even in the face of danger to the public."[30]

Other Driving Issues in Epilepsy

Some physicians may advise controlled seizure patients not to drive while or after discontinuing antiepileptic (AED) medications.[6,18] However, only one state in the United

States (Maine) actually has rules that require such restriction.[16] Still, it seems prudent for physicians to advise or warn patients with epilepsy who are driving about the increased risk of seizure occurrence when medications are reduced or stopped.[31] One AED withdrawal study prospectively followed patients with epilepsy who were in remission for at least 2 years. The recurrence risk for these patients was 30% over 12 months following AED withdrawal. Among those who were seizure-free for 3 months following AED discontinuation, the subsequent 12-month seizure recurrence risk was 15%, and for those who were seizure-free for 6 months, that risk was 9%.[32] If seizures recur after AEDs are discontinued, several states make special allowance for early resumption of driving privileges once medications are restarted.[16,18]

In the United States, state rules regarding driving for patients who have had a single seizure are generally not distinguished from those for epilepsy.[16,18,33] However, in the United Kingdom, individuals who experience a single unprovoked seizure are officially allowed to regain ordinary driving privileges after a shorter seizure-free interval (6 months) than individuals with established epilepsy or recurrent seizures (12 months).[25] Unprovoked seizures are defined as seizures not due to an acute precipitating cause such as a stroke, head trauma, or infection.[33] The United Kingdom guidelines specifically aim to allow driving for individuals with a first unprovoked seizure who have a less than 20% risk of experiencing a recurrent seizure in the next year.[25] A recent prospective study of Australian adults with a first-time seizure proposed 2.5% as an acceptable monthly risk for seizure recurrence and found that for the monthly risk of seizure recurrence to fall within that range a seizure-free period of 8 months before licensure would be required.[26]

Certain clinical factors increase the risk of seizure recurrence after a single unprovoked seizure, including having a known brain lesion as the cause of the seizure (a remote symptomatic seizure), an epileptiform abnormality on the electroencephalogram, a significant abnormality on brain imaging, or a nocturnal seizure.[33] Evidence also indicates that early drug treatment reduces the risk of seizure recurrence, particularly within the first 2 years after a first seizure, when the risk of recurrence is greatest.[33] Regulatory authorities may take into account whether a patient is taking AEDs when determining whether or when to permit licensure to drive after a first seizure. For example, one study reported that patients with single unprovoked seizures who were treated with AEDs early were more likely to be driving at 2-year follow-up.[34] A provoked seizure is one that is caused by an acute illness or related to an isolated event, such as hypoglycemia, which is unlikely to recur. In general, a provoked seizure has a lower risk of recurrence than an unprovoked seizure, so they may warrant less severe restrictions regarding driving.

Physicians who care for individuals with epilepsy are involved in the diagnosis and management of patients with psychogenic nonepileptic seizures (PNES). Although PNES is not epilepsy, the events mimic epileptic seizures, and patients with PNES generally are not able to predict or control these episodes. Driving risks for individuals with PNES are reported to be low.[35] Although some experts report recommending no driving restrictions for individuals with PNES, the majority either endorse restrictions similar to those for epilepsy or decide on an individualized case-by-case basis.[35–37]

Clinicians have an important role in evaluating the abilities and risks for patients with seizure disorders for driving. However, clinicians must remember that they neither grant nor suspend driving privileges; this is the sole legal prerogative of the state. Physicians should counsel patients regarding the risks associated with driving and epilepsy and the applicable driving laws in their state. The EF is a good resource for the most updated state-specific rules on driving and epilepsy to which patients can be directed. Clinicians should offer information about alternatives to driving for individuals with seizures who will not be permitted to drive. This information concerning alternatives to driving should include information about public transportation and state and local resources for transportation for people with disabilities, including seizures and epilepsy. Local EF affiliates and the national EF are potential resources for this type of information at: http://www.epilepsyfoundation.org/resources/drivingandtravel.cfm.

One fascinating and rapidly evolving field that may offer exciting alternatives for individuals with seizures or other disabilities who not are allowed or able to drive is the self-driving or so-called autonomous driving car. This concept is in active development by several major companies and may become a viable solution for many of the problems relating to epilepsy and driving.[38]

COMMERCIAL DRIVING RULES

In the United States, commercial driving restrictions for people with seizures or epilepsy differ from those pertaining to personal vehicles. Commercial driving restrictions for people with seizures or epilepsy are stricter than those pertaining to private motor vehicle use. In the United States, regulations regarding commercial vehicles involved in intrastate commerce vary among individual states. In general, they do not govern cab drivers, chauffeurs, or drivers of vehicles potentially carrying less than a specified number of individuals, or of less than a specified weight. Individual state rules govern such drivers and vary but generally require only a standard state license. Individual state rules can be found on a useful online Web site, www.dmv.org/special-licenses.php, and through specific state regulatory agencies. Individually, states are increasing implementing standards for intrastate commercial driving that are consistent with the federal government standards for interstate commercial driving. Many states have specific regulations governing school bus or other bus drivers.

Federal regulations up until April 2014 specifically prohibited interstate commercial driving by any person with epilepsy or any person taking AEDs. These standards have recently been modified to follow the slightly less strict recommendations of a 2007 expert panel. They now allow exceptions for some people with well-controlled epilepsy to drive commercial vehicles even if they are still taking AEDs.[39] For example, the new standard specifies that to be licensed: "Individual must have been seizure free for a minimum of 8 years on or off anti-seizure medication; and if all anti-seizure medications have been stopped, the individual must have been seizure free for minimum of 8 years from the time of medication cessation; or if still using anti-seizure medication, the individual must have been on a stable medication regime for a minimum of 2 years. An individual with a history of epilepsy who has been granted conditional certification to drive a commercial motor vehicle must be recertified on an annual basis."[39] People who experience a seizure caused by a known medical condition, such as an acute infection or metabolic disturbance (acute symptomatic seizure), are deferred from licensure as commercial drivers until they are fully recovered from that condition and have no significant residual complications.[39] These new rules and regulations can be found[39] in the Federal Register along with preliminary information on how they will be implemented.[40] Several other countries have different rules and regulations for commercial drivers. As an example, in the United Kingdom, the law prohibits any person who has suffered an epileptic attack since the age of 5 years from driving a heavy or public service vehicle.[41]

EMPLOYMENT

Employment is a major concern and problem for people with seizures.[1,3,4] Epilepsy differs from many other disabilities in that it is episodic and often not apparent to others. This relative invisibility of epilepsy may account for a lack of attention it gets as a barrier to employment. Indeed, surveys indicate that epilepsy is the medical disability considered least favorably by prospective employers.[42] Unemployment rates for people with epilepsy in the United States vary from 12% to 50%, depending on the frequency and type of seizure disorder and associated medical, psychological, and social problems.[43,44] These problems with employment pose major difficulties for patients with epilepsy, their families, and society as a whole. For example, the annual cost attributed to epilepsy in the United States in 1995 is estimated to be $12.5 billion[45] and consists primarily of the lost productivity caused by unemployment and underemployment for patients with intractable or uncontrolled seizures (**Fig. 3**).[45] Underemployment refers to those people who are employed but occupy positions of a lower grade than is warranted by their aptitude.[42–45]

Misconceptions and prejudices about people with epilepsy also contribute to these employment problems. Current social and legal trends aim to combat discrimination against people with medical disabilities such as epilepsy and bring down barriers to employment. Most people with epilepsy are capable of functioning at a high level, with about 50% of those with newly diagnosed epileptic seizures controlled completely with medications, while an additional 20% to 30% achieve seizure control that is adequate for functioning without major limitations.[1,45]

Physicians, and especially neurologists and occupational physicians, are often involved with this issue of employment and seizures. Physicians may serve as advisors to patients, employers, or regulatory agencies. They may be asked to comment on the appropriateness of a particular profession or job for someone with seizures. Doctors need to consider the specific manifestations of a patient's seizures in relation to functional requirements of a particular job to properly counsel patients.

US federal regulations have opened more employment opportunities for those with disabilities such as epilepsy; this is important to communicate to both patients and employers. The Americans with Disabilities Act (ADA), a federal law passed in 1990, confers civil rights protection by law on people with disabilities such as epilepsy. These rights are similar to those provided on the basis of race, sex, national origin,

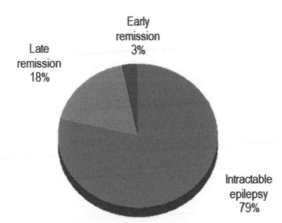

Fig. 3. The great majority of societal costs related to epilepsy (amounting to $12.5 billion in 1995) are related to unemployment, underemployment, and reduced productivity in individuals with intractable epilepsy and seizures. (*Data from* Begley CE, Famulari M, Annegers JF, et al. The cost of epilepsy in the United States: an estimate from population based clinical and survey data. Epilepsia 2000;41:342–51.)

or religion.[46,47] In July 2004, employment guidelines were released by the Equal Employment Opportunity Commission (EEOC), a US federal agency providing support for patients with epilepsy in the workplace.[3,48]

The ADA specifically prohibits discrimination against qualified people with disabilities in employment, public services and transportation, public accommodations, and telecommunications services.[1,47,48] Importantly, the ADA does not invalidate or limit the rights or remedies provided by federal, state, or local laws that may confer greater protection than the ADA. The ADA covers employers with 15 or more employees. Although some employers may be excluded, they are likely covered by similar federal or state antidiscrimination regulations.

STANDARDS FOR EMPLOYMENT

Most jobs are suitable for people with epilepsy. Blanket or categorical prohibitions should be avoided and are usually not legal in the United States. When medical advice is sought about the suitability of particular jobs for people with epilepsy, the guidance given should take into account the requirements of the job and the known facts about epilepsy and seizures. The organization of the work practice should be examined by the employer for jobs associated with a high physical risk to the individual worker or to others in an effort to reduce this potential risk to an acceptable level. Only in those situations in which such risk reduction cannot be achieved are restrictions on the employment of people with epilepsy justified.

The ADA defines a disability as a physical or mental impairment that substantially limits one or more of the major life activities as determined by functions such as caring for oneself, performing manual tasks, walking, seeing, hearing, speaking, breathing, learning, and working. Epilepsy is historically and legally considered a disability that substantially limits life activities, especially when it is not controlled.[47,48]

The provisions of the ADA are regularly reinterpreted and modified by specific court rulings. Recent interpretations by the EEOC have expanded the definition of epilepsy as a disability to include "limitations that occur as the result of seizures or because of side effects or complications that can result from medications used to control the condition." In addition, the expanded designation now allows persons with epilepsy to qualify for disability if the seizures have substantially limited the person's activities for some time in the past (before the seizures were controlled) or if the employer treats the individual as if the epilepsy significantly affects the person's life activities.[48] Under the ADA, people with disabilities should not be excluded from employment opportunities unless they are actually unable to perform the job. Consequently, categorical prohibitions of employment of people with epilepsy in any profession, which were previously widespread, are now illegal for most employers.

Several studies have also shown that the disability conferred by epilepsy is not only a result of the seizures and medications but also due to common comorbidities, including cognitive or motor impairment and mood disorders, such as depression and anxiety. These concomitant disorders can significantly affect quality of life in patients with epilepsy and impact social and vocational factors as well as overall disability.[49,50]

The ADA also requires employers to make "reasonable accommodations" for the known physical or mental limitations of a qualified person with a disability, unless to do so would impose an "undue hardship." "Reasonable accommodation" refers to any change in the work environment or the way tasks are customarily performed that enables a person with a disability to experience equal employment opportunities. "Undue hardship" refers to changes that would be difficult or expensive to implement.

However, employers may also be legally justified in requiring that an employee should not pose a direct threat of substantial imminent risk to the health or safety of other people in the workplace.[45,46]

International guidelines for employment of people with epilepsy have also been developed.[51] These guidelines propose the following:

- Neither the diagnosis of epilepsy nor the actual occurrence of seizures should discourage a person from paid employment.
- In most instances in which restrictions on particular types of employment are necessary, such decisions must be based on fair and individual assessments of both the demands of the work chosen and the people with epilepsy concerned, otherwise such restrictions are discriminatory.
- All people with epilepsy should have equal opportunities in gaining access to available health care and rehabilitation as well as vocational programs and social support services to gain maximal control over their disorder and to maximize their chances of employment.
- In regard to job seeking, selection, and employment, people with epilepsy should be endowed with the same rights as other workers.

SAFETY AND PREVENTION

For jobs with a higher physical risk to the worker or others, the details of the work should be examined, and there should be efforts on the part of the employer to reduce this danger to an acceptable level. Only when such risk reduction cannot be achieved are restrictions on the employment justified and potentially legal. The ADA specifically prohibits exclusion of qualified people with epilepsy from employment opportunities unless they are actually unable to perform the job. Categorical prohibitions of employment of people with epilepsy in any capacity are now illegal for most employers and for almost all jobs except for a few such as mentioned in later discussion.

Jobs or Careers with Epilepsy or Seizure-Specific Standards and Restrictions:

- Commercial driver (eg, for interstate driving and federal licensure)
- Airplane pilot
- Bus driver
- Military service
- Law enforcement officers (rules vary by state)

Accident risk is a major consideration in employment decisions. In general, although people with epilepsy have a somewhat higher overall accident rate, injuries provoked by work accidents are generally mild and unrelated to seizures.[52,53] In studies of employers of people with epilepsy, seizure-related work accidents and absence rates are not reported as substantial problems for people with epilepsy.[52–55] Indeed, it can be said that for people with epilepsy, it is not work that is dangerous, but it is their epilepsy and seizures. Individuals with epilepsy are exposed to the risks of seizure in their daily lives regardless of whether they are at work, at home, or in the community. Most people with epilepsy are actually capable of functioning and succeeding at a high level. After someone with active seizures begins work, it may be advisable for that person to inform selected coworkers of the problem, so that panic and other inappropriate responses to seizures are avoided. When seizures are likely in the workplace, education of coworkers and supervisors may help avoid or deal with misunderstandings. The EF (http://www.epilepsy.com) has specific resources to help with employment and legal support.

SELECTED ISSUES IN THE EMPLOYMENT OF PEOPLE WITH EPILEPSY

Some companies require a pre-employment health screening and physical examination. However, many laws prohibit broad inquiries into an applicant's past medical history unless it pertains to the actual performance of a specific job. In the United States, a person is not legally obliged to offer medical information that is not relevant to the performance of a specific job. When a person's epilepsy has direct bearing on the performance of a job, then he or she is legally required to answer questions about the disability.[47]

Potential illegal discrimination against people with disabilities such as epilepsy can be avoided by offering positions or jobs on the basis of qualifications before requiring a medical history, physical examination, or drug screening. After the job is offered, the decision as to whether the applicant is able to perform the responsibilities of the position can be made without preference or discrimination.

The ADA specifies that an employer may ask a potential employee whether he or she is able to perform job-related functions with or without reasonable accommodations. In addition, the employer may ask an applicant to describe or demonstrate how he or she would perform specific job duties. However, the employer is not permitted to ask whether the potential employee has a disability or to inquire about the severity of such a disability.[47]

For people with seizures who are having difficulties with employment, vocational rehabilitation should be considered. Some studies demonstrate that it can be beneficial in aiding people with epilepsy achieve successful competitive employment in the community.[44,56–58] Seizure control is a predictor of successful rehabilitation and job placement.[44,56]

EPILEPSY AND MILITARY SERVICE

The US military services use epilepsy as a categorical restriction for enlistment, and despite legal protections against discrimination in general employment, the armed services are essentially exempt and exclude people with epilepsy. The rationale given is that the military requires its members to be available for worldwide service on an emergency basis and in areas with limited or absent medical facilities or personnel. Regulations generally require that an applicant to any military service be considered on an individual basis, but still require that there have been no seizures since the age of 5, or that the applicant has been seizure-free without medication for the 5 years before the application. Further information on this is available at: http://www.epilepsy.com/get-help/managing-your-epilepsy/independent-living/employment/safety-sensitive-jobs/military-service.

Should someone already enlisted in the military develop a seizure of epilepsy, the standards may be more lenient. Medication use may be permitted, but complete seizure control and seizure freedom is still the required standard for retention. Decisions are made on an individualized basis that may vary with the service branch.

EPILEPSY AND FEDERAL DISABILITY BENEFITS

Sometimes people with epilepsy are just not able to work because of their seizures or related medical disabilities and may therefore want or need to apply for government disability benefits. Physicians participate extensively in this process by counseling patients on qualifications for disability and by informing authorities about their patients' disabilities. In addition, some physicians may also serve as reviewers or advisors for the Social Security Administration to determine or make recommendations regarding a patient's eligibility and benefits. The eligibility criteria for federal disability benefits within the US social security system are strict and the process for establishing disability is complex, based on rather arbitrary standards, and not always equitable. This information is available online.[59]

In the social security system, disability is defined as the inability to engage in substantial gainful activity by reason of any medically determinable physical or mental impairment that can be expected to result in death or that has lasted or can be expected to last for a continuous period of not less than 12 months. Moreover, for a person to qualify for disability benefits, the impairment must be of such severity that, taking into account the person's age, education, and work experience, he or she is unable to do the same work as previously or to participate in any other substantial gainful activity that exists in the national economy.[56] This condition does not necessarily imply that work is impossible; some people who meet disability requirements still work. However, it is intended to refer to an impairment with which most people would be unable to work.

The specific criteria for federal disability benefits for epilepsy are complex.[59] Requirements for documentation of a disorder and consideration of significant impairment are strictly and rather arbitrarily defined. No scientific studies have confirmed the validity of the specific criteria. The requirements for meeting the epilepsy "listing" or designation specify the following:

- Provision of a detailed description of a typical seizure (given by a physician or other reliable observer)
- Impairment despite adherence to prescribed antiepileptic treatment (determination of the blood concentration of antiepileptic therapy may indicate compliance)
- The degree of impairment will be determined according to type, frequency, duration, and sequelae of seizures

Factors that determine that the severity of the condition is sufficient for a person with convulsive (grand mal or psychomotor) epilepsy to qualify for disability benefits include the following:

- A seizure frequency equal to or greater than once a month
- The persistence of seizures despite treatment for 3 months or longer
- Diurnal (daytime) episodes with loss of consciousness and convulsive seizures or nocturnal (nighttime) episodes that manifest residuals that interfere significantly with daytime activity

For a person with nonconvulsive epilepsy (petit mal, psychomotor, or focal), those factors include the following:

- A seizure frequency equal to or greater than once a week
- The persistence of seizures despite 3 months or more of treatment
- Seizures that result in alteration of consciousness or loss of consciousness, transient postictal manifestations of unconventional behavior, or significant interference with daytime activity[34]

These rules are rather arbitrary and present various problems. For example, the blood concentration of AEDs is only one indication of compliance with treatment. Blood concentration is also not as important an indicator of treatment efficacy for many of the newer antiepileptic agents as it is for older medications such as phenytoin.

In addition, if a person does not meet these requirements, other criteria may be considered when determining whether that person has a disability that is functionally equivalent to an approved listing.[59] These criteria include the following:

- Average seizure frequency
- Seizure severity
- Combination of impairments such as developmental delay, intellectual disability, psychological deficits, motor or other neurologic disorders, and drug effects on cognition and behavior.

These standards are in some respect redundant, not entirely clear, and remain open to varied interpretations.

Last, the social security disability system is structured in such a way that initial applications are much more likely to be refused than are subsequent appeals. Initial denials are relatively routine, and persistence is often rewarded. Some patients benefit from assistance from lawyers who specialize in this type of action and who will work for contingency fees, which is an advantage for patients with limited resources. The amounts of money concerned in the award of benefits can be substantial because payments are retroactive and based on the date at which the person was first established to have become disabled.

The legal resources available to people with epilepsy or seizures who need assistance with legal or regulatory issues are varied. For people of adequate means, private attorneys are available for almost all areas of need. Some lawyers specialize in specific issues, such as federal disability cases. Appropriate private lawyers can be identified through bar referral services or through the national Legal Advocacy Department or local affiliates of the EF. Every state also has consumer protection and advocacy groups to assist people with epilepsy and other disabilities. These agencies are federally funded and mandated services, and they can be identified by contacting state or federal resources or through the national office, local affiliates of the EF or their Web site. Some of these agencies provide direct legal services, whereas others have a comprehensive referral network.

All states and many local jurisdictions also have a legal aid program for low-income people who qualify. Such programs can help people involved in noncriminal matters. Public defenders are available for people of limited means who are implicated in criminal matters.

REFERENCES

1. IOM (Institute of Medicine). Epilepsy across the spectrum: promoting health and understanding. Washington, DC: The National Academies Press; 2012.
2. Temkin O. The falling sickness. 2nd edition. Baltimore (MD): The Johns Hopkins Press; 1971.
3. Gilliam F, Kuzniecky R, Faught E, et al. Patient-validated content of epilepsy-specific quality-of-life measurement. Epilepsia 1997;38:233–6.
4. Moran NF, Poole K, Bell G, et al. Epilepsy in the United Kingdom: seizure frequency and severity, anti-epileptic drug utilization and impact on life in 1652 people with epilepsy. Seizure 2004;13:425–33.
5. Gilliam F, Hecimovic H, Sheline Y. Psychiatric comorbidity, health, and function in epilepsy. Epilepsy Behav 2003;4(Suppl 4):26–30.
6. Krumholz A, Fisher RS, Lesser RP, et al. Driving and epilepsy: a review and reappraisal. JAMA 1991;265:622–6.
7. Krumholz A. Driving issues in epilepsy: past, present, and future. Current review in clinical science. Epilepsy Curr 2009;9:31–5.

8. Edmondstone WM. How do we manage the first seizure in adults? J R Coll Physicians Lond 1995;29:289–94.

9. Drazkowski JF, Neiman ES, Sirven JL, et al. Frequency of physician counseling and attitudes toward driving motor vehicles in people with epilepsy: comparing a mandatory-reporting with a voluntary-reporting state. Epilepsy Behav 2010; 19:52–4.

10. Sheth SG, Krauss G, Krumholz A, et al. Mortality in epilepsy: driving fatalities vs. other causes of death in patients with epilepsy. Neurology 2004;63: 1002–7.

11. Waller JA. Chronic medical conditions and traffic safety. N Engl J Med 1965;273: 1413–20.

12. Hansiota P, Broste SK. The effect of epilepsy or diabetes on the risk of automobile accidents. N Engl J Med 1991;324:22–6.

13. Taylor J, Chadwick D, Johnson T. Risks of accidents in drivers with epilepsy. J Neurol Neurosurg Psychiatry 1996;60:621–7.

14. Crancer A Jr, McMurray L. Accident and violation rates in Washington's medically restricted drivers. JAMA 1968;205:74–9.

15. Masland RL. The physician's responsibility for epileptic drivers. Ann Neurol 1978; 4:485–6.

16. Krauss GK, Ampaw L, Krumholz A. Individual state driving restrictions for people with epilepsy in the US. Neurology 2001;57:1780–5.

17. Krauss GK, Krumholz A, Carter RC, et al. Risk factors for seizure-related motor vehicle crashes in patients with epilepsy. Neurology 1999;52:1324–9.

18. Anonymous. Consensus statements, sample statutory provisions, and model regulations regarding driver licensing and epilepsy. American Academy of Neurology. American Epilepsy Society, Epilepsy Foundation of America. Epilepsia 1994;35:696–705.

19. Berg AT, Vickrey BG, Sperling MR, et al. Driving in adults with refractory localization-related epilepsy. Multi-Center Study of Epilepsy Surgery. Neurology 2000;54(3):625–30.

20. Dalrymple J, Appleby J. Cross sectional study of reporting of epileptic seizures to general practitioners. BMJ 2000;320(7227):94–7.

21. van der Lugt PJM. Is an application form useful to select patients with epilepsy who may drive? Epilepsia 1975;16:743–6.

22. Gastaut H, Zifkin BG. The risk of automobile accidents with seizures occurring while driving: relation to seizure type. Neurology 1987;37:1613–6.

23. Drazkowski JF, Fisher RS, Sirven JI, et al. Seizure-related motor vehicle crashes in Arizona before and after reducing the driving restriction from 12 to 3 months. Mayo Clin Proc 2003;78:819.

24. Fisher RS, Parsonage M, Beaussart M, et al. Epilepsy and driving: an international perspective. Epilepsia 1994;35:675–84.

25. Bonnet LJ, Tudur-Smith C, Williamson PR, et al. Risk of recurrence after a first seizure and implications for driving: further analysis of the multicentre study of early epilepsy and single seizures. BMJ 2010;341:c6477.

26. Brown JWL, Lawn ND, Lee J, et al. When is it safe to return to driving after a first-ever seizure? J Neurol Neurosurg Psychiatry 2015;86:60–4.

27. Bacon D, Fisher RS, Morris JC, et al. American Academy of Neurology position statement on physician reporting of medical conditions that may affect driving competence. Neurology 2007;68:1174–7.

28. McLachlan RS, Starreveld E, Lee MA. Impact of mandatory physician reporting on accident risk in epilepsy. Epilepsia 2007;48:1500–5.

29. Redelmeier DA, Christopher J, Yarnell AB, et al. Physicians' warnings for unfit drivers and the risk of trauma from road crashes. N Engl J Med 2012;367: 1228–36.
30. Black L. Physicians' responsibility to report impaired drivers. AMA Journal of Ethics (Formerly, Virtual Mentor) 2008;10:393–6.
31. Quality Standards Subcommittee of the American Academy of Neurology. Practice parameter: a guideline for discontinuing antiepileptic drugs in seizure-free patients. Neurology 1996;47:600–2.
32. Bonnett LJ, Shukralla A, Tudur-Smith C, et al. Seizure recurrence after antiepileptic drug withdrawal and the implications for driving: further results from the Medical Research Council Antiepileptic Drug Withdrawal Study and a systematic review. J Neurol Neurosurg Psychiatry 2011;82:1328–33.
33. Krumholz A, Wiebe S, Gronseth GS, et al. Evidence-based guideline: management of an unprovoked first seizure in adults: report of the guideline development subcommittee of the American Academy of Neurology and the American Epilepsy Society. Neurology 2015;84:1705–13.
34. Jacoby A, Gamble C, Doughty J, et al, Medical Research Council MESS Study Group. Quality of life outcomes of immediate or delayed treatment of early epilepsy and single seizures. Neurology 2007;68:1188–96.
35. Benbadis SR, Blustein JN, Sunstad L. Should patients with psychogenic nonepileptic seizures be allowed to drive? Epilepsia 2000;41:895–7.
36. Specht U, Thorbecke R. Should patients with psychogenic nonepileptic seizures be allowed to drive? Recommendations of German experts. Epilepsy Behav 2009;16:547–50.
37. Morrison I, Razvi SSM. Driving regulations and psychogenic non-epileptic seizures: perspectives from the United Kingdom. Epilepsy Behav 2011;20: 177–80.
38. Cyrus P. How autonomous vehicle policy in California and Nevada addresses technological and non-technological liabilities. Intersect Stanford J Sci Technol Soc 2012;5:1–16.
39. Engel J, Fisher RS, Krauss GL, et al. Expert panel recommendations: seizure disorders and commercial motor vehicle driver safety. FMCSA. Available at: www.fmcsa. dot.gov/sites/fmcsa.dot.gov/files/docs/Seizure-Disorders-MEP-Recommendations-v2-prot.pdf. Accessed October 15, 2007.
40. Federal Register. Qualification of drivers—exemptions epilepsy and seizure disorders 2014. Available at: https://www.federalregister.gov/articles/2014/04/25/2014-09447/qualification-of-drivers-exemption-applications-epilepsy-and-seizure-disorders.
41. Ooi WW, Gutrecht JA. International regulations for automobile driving and epilepsy. J Travel Med 2000;7:1–4.
42. Hicks MJ, Hicks RA. Attitudes of major employers toward the employment of people with epilepsy: a 30-year study. Epilepsia 1991;32:86–8.
43. Frazier RT, Clemmons D, Trejo W, et al. Program evaluation in epilepsy rehabilitation. Epilepsia 1983;24:734–46.
44. Chaplin JE, Wester A, Tomson T. Factors associated with employment problems of people with established epilepsy. Seizure 1998;7:299–303.
45. Begley CE, Famulari M, Annegers JF, et al. The cost of epilepsy in the United States: an estimate from population-based clinical and survey data. Epilepsia 2000;41:342–51.
46. Anonymous. Americans with Disabilities Act 1990 (Public Law 101–336). Volume 42 of the United States Code. Section 1201.

47. Costin LO, Feldblum C, Webber DW. Disability discrimination in America. JAMA 1999;281:745–52.
48. Anonymous. Questions and answers about epilepsy in the workplace and the Americans with Disabilities Act (ADA) 2004. US Equal Employment Opportunity Commission. Available at: www.eeoc.gov/facts/epilepsy.html.
49. Gilliam FG. The impact of epilepsy on subjective health status. Curr Neurol Neurosci Rep 2003;3(4):357–62.
50. Gilliam FG, Santos J, Vahle V, et al. Depression in epilepsy: ignoring clinical expression of neuronal network dysfunction? Epilepsia 2004;45(Suppl 2):28–33.
51. International Bureau for Epilepsy's Employment Commission. Employing people with epilepsy: principles for good practice. Epilepsia 1989;30:411–2.
52. Dasgutpa AK, Saunders M, Dick DJ. Epilepsy in the British Steel Corporation: an evaluation of sickness, accident and work records. Br J Ind Med 1982;39:145–8.
53. Beghi E, Cornaggia C. Morbidity and accidents in patients with epilepsy: results of a European cohort study. Epilepsia 2002;43:1076–83.
54. Palmer KT, D'Angelo S, Harris EC, et al. Epilepsy, diabetes mellitus and accidental injury at work. Occup Med 2014;64:448–53.
55. Cornaggia CM, Beghi M, Moltrasio L, et al. Accidents at work among people with epilepsy. Results of a European prospective cohort study. Seizure 2006;15:313–9.
56. Freeman JM, Gayle E. Rehabilitation and the client with epilepsy: a survey of the client's view of the rehabilitation process and its results. Epilepsia 1978;19:233–9.
57. Carroll D. Employment among young people with epilepsy. Seizure 1992;1:12–131.
58. Bautista RE, Shapovalov E, Saada F, et al. The societal integration of individuals with epilepsy: perspectives for the 21st century. Epilepsy Behav 2014;35:42–9.
59. Official Social Security Website. Disability Professionals Blue Book—Neurological Adults. Available at: http://ssa.gov/disability/professionals/bluebook/11.00-Neurological-Adult.

Patient Education

Identifying Risks and Self-Management Approaches for Adherence and Sudden Unexpected Death in Epilepsy

Patricia Osborne Shafer, RN, MN[a,b,*], Jeffrey Buchhalter, MD, PhD[c]

KEYWORDS

- Patient education • Epilepsy • Sudden unexpected death in epilepsy • SUDEP
- Epilepsy self-management • Adherence

KEY POINTS

- Patient education in epilepsy is one part of quality epilepsy care and is an evolving and growing field of its own.
- Although there may be many barriers to providing appropriate and effective education in some settings, there are even more compelling reasons to educate patients and their families.
- Health outcomes, patient satisfaction, safety, patient/provider communication, and quality of life may all be affected by what people are taught (or not taught), what they understand, and how they use this information to make decisions and manage their health.
- Data regarding learning needs and interventions to address medication adherence and sudden unexpected death in epilepsy education can be used to guide clinicians in health care or community settings.
- Ideally, clinicians can enhance their individual educational efforts by encouraging the use of credible community and online information and resources to improve access to epilepsy information and support.

INTRODUCTION

Educating patients and families is a critical component of quality epilepsy care. Effective education takes time, which can be a barrier for clinicians providing care in some settings. Additionally, changing concepts in our understanding of epilepsy, comorbidities, risks, and response to treatment have complicated how and what to teach

[a] Beth Israel Deaconess Medical Center, 330 Brookline Avenue KS 457, Boston, MA 02215, USA;
[b] Epilepsy Foundation, Landover, MD 20785-2353, USA; [c] Comprehensive Children's Epilepsy Centre, Alberta Children's Hospital, Cumming School of Medicine, University of Calgary, 2888 Shaganappi Trail Northwest, Calgary, Alberta T3B 6A8, Canada
* Corresponding author. Beth Israel Deaconess Medical Center, 330 Brookline Avenue KS 457, Boston, MA 02215.
E-mail address: pshafe@comcast.net

Neurol Clin 34 (2016) 443–456
http://dx.doi.org/10.1016/j.ncl.2016.01.001
0733-8619/16/$ – see front matter
neurologic.theclinics.com

people, but also highlight the importance of patient education. This article discusses goals and priorities for patient education and how learning and self-management needs may vary across the spectrum and along an individual's journey with epilepsy. Evidence and best practices for 2 major areas, medication adherence and sudden unexpected death in epilepsy (SUDEP), are highlighted.

GOALS OF PATIENT EDUCATION AND SELF-MANAGEMENT

Providing information to people with epilepsy and families aims to increase knowledge and understanding of epilepsy and the specific topic(s) addressed (eg, medication, adherence, seizure types, safety, first aid). However, numerous studies and trends in education show that providing information and increasing knowledge by itself does not necessarily affect clinical outcomes or influence how a person is able to use the information to manage their epilepsy.

Epilepsy self-management education takes this a step further. Self-management concepts and approaches stress the active involvement of the person with epilepsy, family, or other caregiver with their health care team. The concept of epilepsy self-management has evolved from addressing the steps or processes needed for a person to control their epilepsy and effects of having epilepsy[1] to a focus on ways to "optimize seizure control, minimize the effects of having a seizure disorder, and to maximize quality of life in partnership with their health care provider".[2] These approaches strive to change a person's behavior and promote healthy behaviors rather than just increase knowledge. Teaching skills, building self-efficacy, and providing resources and support for people to apply the learned information to their management needs are critical aspects of self-management education.[3] Ideally the clinician works together with the patient to identify learning needs and priorities and how best to meet their needs.

The importance of patient-centered care and education was emphasized in the landmark publication, Crossing the Quality Chasm: A New Health System for the 21st Century, and is a critical factor in a model for organization and integration of care and services for people with epilepsy.[4] This epilepsy care model acknowledges that people receive care in many different settings and that both health care facilities and community supports are part of the patient's care team. Patient-centered care is at the heart of the model and ideally leads to informed and engaged patients/families working collaboratively with their health care team and community supports. This epilepsy care model assumes that patient education and self-management support occur across settings and are part of care leading to optimal outcomes and family adaptation.

CORE COMPONENTS FOR EPILEPSY EDUCATION

Many models or self-management programs focus primarily on core components to improve epilepsy management, such as managing seizures, treatments, safety, and lifestyle.[1,3,5-7] Yet epilepsy can have wide-reaching ramifications on the health of many, causing or being associated with comorbid conditions such as mood, sleep disorders, mobility, or bone health, to name a few. Epilepsy, particularly when seizures are not controlled or comorbid conditions are present, can affect one's social situation and ability to live independently. In these situations, epilepsy self-management should also address management of general health, comorbid conditions, psychosocial issues, and independent living factors, such as education, employment, living situations, finances, and other disability-related needs that affect a person's ability to live to their fullest.[8]

Thus, self-management education for people with epilepsy can most easily be thought of in 2 parts: epilepsy-specific self-management and chronic care management.[4] Epilepsy-specific self-management addresses the key behaviors needed to optimize epilepsy management, whereas chronic care management focuses more broadly on wellness or maintaining a healthy lifestyle, developing active partnerships, communicating with the health care team, and living independently (**Table 1**).

OUTCOMES OF EDUCATION AND SELF-MANAGEMENT INTERVENTIONS

Outcomes of patient education and self-management can be difficult to assess and generalize because of research methodology used. Reviews of self-management programs or interventions have found varied results from different types of programs.[2,9–11] The review by Edward and colleagues[9] of 14 self-management interventions found that the programs improved knowledge and self-efficacy and impacted psychosocial variables, quality of life, and seizure control. Shafer's[10] review suggested that use of cognitive behavioral approaches seemed to enhance educational programs with skill development. Programs that offered more than a 1- or 2-time intervention tended to have greater impact on seizure control, whereas psychosocial interventions addressed critical comorbidities and affected other behavioral variables important in changing health behaviors.

LEARNING NEEDS AND PRIORITIES

Educational needs of patients and families can vary greatly depending on several variables. Personal variables may include age, gender, and age at seizure onset. Developmental level and cognition are critical aspects that may influence how and what people may need and who should be involved in the educational process. Sociocultural variables such as where the patient lives, cultural beliefs, transportation, financial resources, and health insurance may affect their access to health care and type of services available or used. Many epilepsy variables must be considered for their influence on a person's learning needs and care such as type and severity of seizures and epilepsy syndrome, prognosis, type and response to treatment, adverse events, and comorbid conditions.

Perceptions of learning needs may also vary among a patient, family, and clinician. For example, a person who has lost a job because of a seizure at work may want to focus first on job hunting, addressing perceived discrimination, or the challenges of being unable to drive. Yet the health care provider may recognize the impact of poor seizure control on the person's ability to work safely or want to assess if medication side effects or other factors were contributing factors. All these issues are relevant, but the question arises: where should teaching start?

Examples of Learning Needs

A literature review conducted as part of the Institute of Medicine recommendations for epilepsy highlights some general educational needs for any person with epilepsy (**Box 1**). Different age groups may have additional concerns or needs that focus on age-related needs or risks. For example, needs of children with epilepsy will include common learning problems, educational needs, social skills and relationships, disclosure, lifestyle, mental health, and transition issues. Educating older adults should include issues with new-onset seizures; medication adherence, drug interactions, and adverse events; mobility and fall risk; and cognition and other comorbidities.[3]

Table 1
Areas of self-management for epilepsy

Epilepsy-Specific Management	Examples of Knowledge and Skills
Seizures	Knowledge—specific seizure types, first aid Skills—recognizing, recording, tracking events; identifying seizure triggers; keeping seizure diary, developing seizure response plan
Medications/treatments	Knowledge—Medication name, dose, possible interactions and side effects, consequences of missed doses, drug-alcohol interactions Skills—Tracking medication intake, tracking medication dose and changes, managing refills, responding to allergic reactions or adverse effects; using rescue therapies
Safety	Knowledge—Risks for injury related to seizures and treatment, strategies for reducing injury, risks for mortality including SUDEP Skills—Assessing risks in environment, modifying environment and lifestyle to reduce risks yet maintaining quality of life, developing safety management plan
Comorbid conditions	Knowledge—Common comorbidities, symptoms, treatments, and management Skills—Recognizing symptoms and relation to epilepsy, knowing when to seek support and treatment, monitoring treatment

Chronic Care Management	Examples of Knowledge and Skills

• Maintaining healthy lifestyle
  ○ Physical activity
  ○ Adequate sleep
  ○ Pleasurable activities
  ○ Physical health
  ○ Emotional health
	Knowledge—How seizures and everyday life interact, importance of healthy lifestyle and behavior, symptoms of unhealthy lifestyle
	Skills—Assessing impact of seizures on daily life and making modifications, developing strategies for maintaining healthy lifestyle, seeking emotional support, coping with stressful situations

Active partnership with health care team	Knowledge—Need for active partnership with health care providers, effective communication strategies Skills—Communicating, problem solving, decision making, self-advocating, goal setting, developing action plans
Independent living	Knowledge—Environmental support, resources, services needed Skills—Assessing and evaluating resources, developing action plans, handling emergencies

Adapted from IOM (Institute of Medicine). Epilepsy across the spectrum: Promoting health and understanding. Washington, DC: The National Academies Press, 2012; with permission.

Box 1
Basic educational needs of all people with epilepsy

- Epilepsy—seizure type, syndrome, causes
- Treatment and management—options, medications, devices, surgery, dietary modifications, side effects, treatment discontinuation, seizure triggers, risk for suicidal ideation associated with medications, other management strategies
- Safety risks—risk assessment, seizure first aid, injury prevention, equipment to prevent injury
- Mortality risks—SUDEP, status epilepticus, seizure-related injury, suicide
- Healthy lifestyle—general health, sleep, fatigue, physical exercise
- Possible comorbidities—mental health, cognitive, neurologic, somatic
- Social concerns—engaging new friends, seizures in social settings, telling others, family burden, stigma, education, employment, independent living
- Emotional response—coping, dealing with fears, stress management
- Available informational and community resources—Websites, state and local resources, Epilepsy Foundation, community agencies, health care providers

Adapted from IOM (Institute of Medicine). Epilepsy across the spectrum: Promoting health and understanding. Washington, DC: The National Academies Press, 2012; with permission.

Setting Priorities

Patient-centered care and self-management education starts by acknowledging different needs and collaborating with the patient/family on setting priorities. Priorities in an office visit may focus first on a person's health and safety and issues that can be most easily addressed by the clinician and patient at the time of the encounter. Yet priority setting should also identify needs that can be met by other health care providers, community caregivers, or advocates. For example, assessing the impact of stigma or discrimination and finding accessible transportation would best be addressed by a caregiver or advocate with skills in independent living, employment, and disability issues. It is important to not ignore those issues that the health care professional does not perceive as a priority or does not feel comfortable addressing. Establishing a plan on how the patient can address these most appropriately will ensure that their needs are being heard and acted on in a timely basis.

Decision-making tools are being developed that can help clinicians assess needs and identify priorities. A self-management tool called *MINDSET* helps clinicians and patients with these tasks during clinic visits.[12] The computer-based program tailors action plans for self-management that can be given to patients at clinic visits and allows ways to monitor progress. The public use website of the Epilepsy Foundation (epilepsy.com) has decision support and self-management tools to enhance patient/provider communication, checklists of learning needs, and forms to tailor and monitor progress and adherence. My Seizure Diary, an electronic seizure diary, is a self-management resource that can assist patients and clinicians to assess a person's progress and needs and can provide valuable information to assist in setting priorities and assessing risks.

WHEN SHOULD EDUCATION BE PROVIDED?

General principles of patient education stress that teaching should not be a one-time activity. Information must be presented in a manner that is easy to understand in a format and language easy to digest, ideally tailored to the individual, and reinforced over time. Yet following these principles can be difficult in an office or clinic setting. The limited amount of time for patient visits and multiple activities that must be accomplished can impede the process. Approaches that may assist clinicians and improve educational outcomes may include:

- Use of checklists to identify patient priorities before visits
- Reinforce verbal teaching with printed literature appropriate to the individual
- Comprehensive clinic visits that allow a nurse to see a patient for assessment and education before or after a physician visit
- Use of electronic medical records and sharing of notes with patients
- Use of credible epilepsy websites that provide information and self-management resources and programs
- Online educational webinars and curricula
- In person, phone, and web-based support groups and mentoring
- Strategies to enhance self-efficacy and support
- Referrals to other health care providers or community agencies to address barriers to education and self-management needs

Timing of education will vary depending on each patient, although there are critical junctures during which all patients should be assessed for their educational needs. These junctures do not all require teaching by a physician or nurse or at a face-to-face visit. Many of these teachable moments may occur during phone calls with nurses and other health care professionals. The Institute of Medicine epilepsy[4] report identified the following examples of critical junctures for patient/family education:

- At diagnosis (many needs begin after first seizure and before diagnosis)
- During first year
- At the time of referral to a specialized epilepsy center
- When there is a change or new concerns develop
  - Developmental status (beginning school, transitions, question of delays)
  - Seizures (breakthrough seizures, type, frequency, clusters, risk for emergencies)
  - Treatment-related concerns (change or stopping medications, surgery, dietary therapy, devices, side effects, adherence, interactions)
  - When treatment fails (reevaluate options)
  - Health status changes (pregnancy, injury, other health complications)
  - Life stressors (moving, change in occupation, change in marital status, death, or grief)
  - Travel (new environments, time changes)
  - Employment and vocational status

In recent years, risks for premature mortality, especially sudden unexpected death in epilepsy (SUDEP) have been highlighted by patients and families as an unmet educational need. The need to address this topic earlier and in a manner that can help people identify and lessen their risks is critical. Additionally, people should recognize and know how to prevent and manage risks for cluster seizures, status epilepticus, injuries, or other adverse events associated with seizures. Unfortunately, these issues are often not discussed until after an untoward event has happened.

Many times, for example, with patients' new-onset seizures, teaching about the diagnosis, care, and treatment is done after the event and, unfortunately, at a time when people may be emotionally overwhelmed. Although this can impede learning for some people, in others the acuity of the situation may enhance their motivation and readiness to learn. It is imperative that clinicians recognize competing influences and consider how much information to provide at the time of diagnosis and provide a mechanism to follow up on retention, understanding, and other concerns that have arisen.

For many topics, teaching should be done proactively. For example, teaching people about seizure triggers and the importance of medication adherence should be done when a medication is prescribed rather than waiting for breakthrough seizures to occur. The importance of folic acid and proper selection of seizure medication should be taught to women of childbearing potential before they become pregnant.

MEDICATION ADHERENCE

Taking medications inconsistently is one of the more common problems that can result in breakthrough seizures or worsening of seizure control. Nonadherence with antiepileptic medications has been documented using retrospective reviews of claims data in 26% of 33,659 patients in a Medicaid population[13,14] and in 39% of 10,892 adults in a managed care population.[15] These studies also found that nonadherence was associated with higher health care use and costs, especially for inpatient and emergency room encounters[14,15] and higher rates of mortality and serious illnesses.[13]

Higher rates of nonadherence have been shown in studies using self-report and medication event monitoring. Cramer and colleagues[16] found that missed doses of seizure medications were reported by 71% of 661 respondents. Seizures after missed doses were reported by 45% of this group. Nonadherence was more likely in people who used seizure medications for longer periods and in drug regimens with greater numbers of daily doses and numbers of tablets taken per day. Other factors that affect medication self-management and adherence include memory difficulties, cost and access to medications, mood, and side effects of medications.

Types of Interventions

Some interventions can be easily delivered by a health care provider, whereas others may be self-administered or provided by other providers or caregivers in health care or community settings. Often, however, clinicians are not aware of what works and what doesn't, and many interventions have not been rigorously evaluated. The following provides examples of educational methods and published results.

Printed drug information

Providing written information about medications is an easy way of teaching patients, but mixed results have been obtained. Interestingly, in Taiwan, 51 adults in an epilepsy clinic were given printed drug information during a clinic visit.[17] Questionnaires were completed before and after the information was provided, including self-reported adherence, and serum drug levels were checked. Knowledge of epilepsy medications improved significantly 1 month after the printed information was given. Self-reported adherence (people who reported being compliant with medications all the time) improved from 74.5% at baseline to 86.3% at follow-up. Forty-one people had drug levels monitored with results within normal ranges and correlating with self-reported adherence.

Combining verbal teaching with printed information and recommending behavioral changes offer the benefit of using multiple modalities. Tang and colleagues[18] compared the effect of providing medication education (verbal and written) that was reinforced by monthly phone calls from a pharmacist with medication education along with a modified medication schedule and behavioral cues. Results found that participants in both groups improved with increased knowledge and adherence to seizure medications, and fewer people had seizures. Adding behavioral cue training did not provide additional benefit in this study.

Structured educational programs

Educational programs provided outside an office or clinic setting have shown improvements in adherence in some studies. For example, Helgeson and colleagues[19] found a reduction in hazardous medical self-management practices, improved compliance by blood levels, and improved seizure control in 39 people who participated in a 2-day psychoeducational program. The effectiveness of a 1-day educational program in Kenya was evaluated in 738 people with epilepsy and their caregivers.[20] People were randomly assigned to an intervention or control group with information collected at baseline and 1 year after the program from 581 people. Blood levels were obtained from 105 people in the intervention group and 86 from a control group but did not show any significant change. Before and after comparisons showed improvement in adherence and seizure control in both groups, yet knowledge about epilepsy improved for people attending the educational intervention. The authors suggested that one-time education did not affect adherence and that repeated efforts may be helpful.

Structured programs offered with multiple sessions have shown benefit on medication adherence. Dash and colleagues[21] developed a structured program in North India that included 4 one-on-one sessions with an epilepsy nurse, each lasting 30 minutes. The intervention consisted of verbal and written information and a phone call follow-up 1 month after participation. Participants were randomly assigned to the educational intervention (N = 82 completed) or usual care (N = 70 completed) and evaluated 6 months after the intervention. Medication adherence increased significantly only in the intervention group. The numbers of people with improved seizure control were significantly greater after the educational program as well.

Pakpour and colleagues[22] also tested a multimodal program in 275 participants with 6-month follow-up. The intervention consisted of 3 in-person meetings (using motivational interviewing approaches, behavior changes to develop adherence plans and address barriers, and self-monitoring) compared with usual care. Again, significant improvements were seen in medication adherence in the educational intervention group compared with the control group.

Self-administered questionnaire

Interventions do not need to be complex. Often just asking about a person's adherence and what they can do to change it may be helpful. Plumpton and colleagues[23] evaluated the impact of a self-administered questionnaire completed after a neurology clinic visit by 61 participants 16 years and older. The intervention asked people questions about medication taking using an "if-then" format. Participants used a Medication Event Monitoring System to monitor adherence over the following month and returned for posttesting. The researchers then estimated the economic impact of the intervention by modeling direct medical costs and health outcomes after matching patients to people with epilepsy in a different long-term trial of seizure medications (Standard and New Antiepileptic Drug) for which the researchers had more extensive data. This modeling approach suggested that the simple questionnaire to assess a person's intent to make behavior changes and take medications can be cost effective.[23]

Online educational self-management program

The Managing Epilepsy Well Network of the Centers for Disease Control has developed eHealth tools that can be easily accessed by people with epilepsy and their families to support and enhance care from the health care team.[2] One of these programs,

WebEase, available through epilepsy.com, is an interactive online self-management program developed using stages of change and motivational interviewing approaches. Three key aspects of self-management are addressed: medication adherence, sleep, and stress. Results of WebEase in a randomized controlled trial of 119 participants showed improvements in one's ability to manage their epilepsy, medication adherence, self-efficacy, sleep quality, and social support.[24,25]

Seizure diaries and reminders

Simple reminders and behavioral cues are frequently used to aid adherence and medication management, especially for people with complex medication regimens or cognitive difficulties. Reminders on cellphones or smartphones, text messaging, and email are examples of interventions that people can implement on their own at no cost. Electronic seizure diaries can send reminders and track medication use, side effects, seizures, and other factors to evaluate the impact of other interventions. Texting4Control, offered by epilepsy.com, is geared to help youth with epilepsy remember medications by sending text messages and tracking medication use.

DISCUSSING SUDEP

Several factors motivate health care providers to educate patients and families including issues that may affect outcome (eg, medication adherence, sleep hygiene, avoidance of alcohol and drugs) and safety (eg, drowning, cooking, operating power tools) and a large category that could be termed *right to know* (eg,. conveying relevant information that will inform prognosis, life planning, and decision making). The rationale for discussing SUDEP with patients and families includes all of these categories. Yet, unfortunately, SUDEP is not talked about often enough, when people feel they need it, or in a manner they can easily understand. Current research addresses discrepancies between what clinicians do or don't do and what families and patients want. The resultant gaps can suggest strategies for improving patient and family education regarding SUDEP. The intent is to prevent SUDEP by encouraging aggressive treatment and adherence.

By 1997, several investigators[26,27] were describing the epidemiology and risk for SUDEP. The definitions suggested were similar, differing mainly on the inclusion or exclusion of the requirement for autopsy to rule out other potential causes of sudden death, primarily cardiac failure and stroke. Subsequently, the definition adopted by many investigators was that offered by Nashef[27]- "...sudden unexpected, non-traumatic and non-drowning death in an individual with epilepsy with or without evidence for a seizure and excluding documented status epilepticus where *post-mortem examination* does not reveal a cause for death." The need for more precise information has led to a unifying definition that classifies cases, based on the amount of data available, into definite, probable, possible, near-SUDEP, and not SUDEP categories.[28] The term *plus* may be added to the above groups when there is a concomitant illness that could have contributed to the sudden death.

Although the reasons for teaching people about SUDEP may seem compelling, articles titled SUDEP: To Discuss or not to Discuss—That Is, the Question[29] and SUDEP: Don't Ask Don't Tell?[30] questioned the wisdom of talking about it. These concerns were raised when SUDEP education had already been incorporated into a national guideline in the United Kingdom. Nonetheless, these thoughtful articles helped spur a productive discussion in the epilepsy community that has helped refine thinking about the topic. An excellent summary of the argument for and against the discussion can be found in the proceedings of a National Institutes of Neurologic Disease and Stroke workshop.[31] The conclusion reached by the participants was that SUDEP should be discussed at some point as part of the general education of all people living with epilepsy and their families unless there are psychological or cultural reasons not to do so.

PROVIDER PREFERENCES FOR SUDEP EDUCATION

There is now a considerable body of literature indicating that most clinicians do not provide SUDEP education most of the time in their interactions with families. One of the earliest studies sent questionnaires to 738 members of the Association of British Neurologists.[30] Of 387 participants (52% response rate), 31% affirmed that they discussed SUDEP with all or most of their patients, whereas 79% indicated that the discussion took place with very few or none of their patients. Slightly better responses were obtained from a survey sent to 250 members of the United Kingdom–based Epilepsy Nurse Association (58% response rate).[32] Half of the nurses indicated that they discussed SUDEP with most of their patients, 6% discussed SUDEP with all patients, whereas 37% discussed it with only a few patients.

A revealing study was performed in a regional pediatric epilepsy clinic in the United Kingdom.[33] Although this is a referral clinic, the types of seizures and epilepsies seen in the clinic are similar to what would be seen in a pediatric epilepsy clinic in the United States and a general pediatric neurology clinic where seizure-related complaints form the majority of most practices. The study design included a survey of 100 consecutive parents and a simultaneous survey sent to 71 pediatric neurologists. Of the pediatric neurologists who responded (65% response rate), 93% indicated that they gave SUDEP information to some of their families, 20% to all, and 63% to people with intractable seizures. Furthermore, 30% believed the information should be given at the time of diagnosis. Perceptions regarding the impact of giving SUDEP information included the following: 35% believed it would improve medication adherence and 41% believed it would increase child supervision.

Similar results about provider preferences for SUDEP education on a routine basis were found in a survey of 315 Italian adult and pediatric neurologists.[34] In response to the statement "I believe that the possibility of a risk of SUDEP should be discussed," only 9% believed it should be discussed with all patients, 20% believed it should be discussed with most, and 62% believed SUDEP should be talked about with very few patients. The reason for discussing SUDEP with 47% of patients was "because of the peculiar status of the disease/treatment." Although not specifically stated, one could infer that this statement refers to specific aspects of an individual's epilepsy care, likely factors associated with intractable seizures.

Regrettably, neurologists in North America did no better than their European colleagues. A recent survey study[35] of 17,588 US and Canadian neurologists (9% returned) found that only 21% of respondents discussed SUDEP 50% of the time or greater, 33% talked about SUDEP 10% to 49% of the time, and 30% rarely talked about it. The most common reasons for not discussing SUDEP were perception of minimal or no risk (53.6%), no proven way to prevent SUDEP (33.8%), impact on quality of life or mood (32.8%), lack of trusting relationship with patient (28.8%), risks of discussion outweigh benefits (25.7%), insufficient time (18.5%), insufficient information about SUDEP (18.3%), not knowing enough about SUDEP (17.8%), and lack of patient support network (15.2%). These reasons fall into 2 broad categories: lack of physician knowledge about what is known about SUDEP and a somewhat paternalistic attitude as to what is best for the patient. The former can be addressed with care provider education and forms the basis of what should be told to people with epilepsy. The latter, although undoubtedly motivated by perception of optimal patient care, requires more of an attitudinal change.

PATIENT AND FAMILY PREFERENCES FOR SUDEP EDUCATION

Responses from people with epilepsy and parents/caregivers paint a different picture. The parents in the study involving the UK pediatric epilepsy referral clinic described above[33] were very clear in their expectations; 91% expected the pediatric neurologist to provide information regarding SUDEP, and 67% wanted this information at the time of diagnosis! The timing of the information was surprising, as it appears to be independent of seizure type or severity. These results stand in direct contrast to what the physicians perceived as the best practice. Additionally, parents responded that the effect of SUDEP disclosure would have a modest effect (30%–50%) on increased supervision, monitoring of medication, and restriction of the child's activities and relatively little effect on the child's and parent's physical, emotional, social, and employment status.

These results were confirmed in a focus group study[36] that included interviews with parents who have a child with mild, moderate, severe, and new-onset epilepsy in addition to a group that lost a child as a result of SUDEP. Qualitative analysis found that all parents wanted SUDEP education, and greater than 50% wanted this information at the first or second visit. Parents also wanted to get the information via face-to-face contact, especially concerning risk assessment and possibilities for prevention.

Adults with epilepsy also want information about SUDEP. Xu and colleagues[37] surveyed 105 adult patients referred to an epilepsy clinic and found that most wanted information about SUDEP. Forty-two percent wanted the education at the first visit and 24% only if seizures worsened. A revealing study of 27 young adults with epilepsy from an epilepsy referral clinic was performed using qualitative analysis of focus group interactions.[38] Similar to the pediatric population, most (81%) believed that information regarding SUDEP should be shared with patients and done at the time of diagnosis. However, only some of the young adults changed their behavior with regard to medication adherence based on that information. Most had a fatalistic attitude as expressed in the title of the publication reporting preliminary results of the study: If You're Going to Die You're Going to Die. This is an important observation, as one of the prime motivators for education is to change behavior, presumably to reduce the risk of seizures and SUDEP.

GENERAL PRACTICES FOR SUDEP EDUCATION: THE WHEN, WHAT AND HOW

Based on this review of the literature, it seems clear that most caregivers of children with epilepsy and those living with epilepsy would like to be educated about SUDEP. People living with epilepsy frequently are misinformed regarding the risks or are unaware of SUDEP. Thus, education should be directed to providing accurate information regarding the occurrence and risk factors relating to SUDEP.[39–42] The factors that place a patient at the highest risk include treatment resistance, generalized tonic clonic seizures that occur during sleep, and a symptomatic etiology. In this group, the purpose of education is to encourage aggressive pursuit of and adherence to treatment (eg, medication, surgery, device or diet).

The "when" of the discussion should ideally occur at the time of the first office visit and as often as necessary to reinforce the necessity of controlling seizures and exploring options to do so. A similar message should be provided to people with other types of motor seizures that occur during wakefulness, as even one generalized tonic clonic seizure per year increases the risk of SUDEP by 3-fold.[43] It should also be noted that SUDEP occurs in those with nonmotor seizures but at a significantly lower rate.

The "what" of the conversation should include general information about the elevated risk of premature mortality in people with epilepsy followed by how this relates to the individual based on their specific risk factors.

The "how" of the education is much more difficult. People differ in how they learn best (eg, direct conversation, printed materials, repetition), and there are many factors (educational, cultural, and emotional backgrounds) that may act as barriers to learning. The shock of hearing that they or a loved one has a potentially life-threatening condition may also influence how people perceive and receive information about SUDEP.

What is the role of education in the lower-risk group, for example, children with non-convulsive seizure with no known etiology and with normal development and neurologic examinations or adults with controlled, nonconvulsive seizures of unknown etiology? Many of these individuals will have heard about SUDEP from a support organization, friends, popular media, or the internet and have unrealistic fears of death associated with epilepsy. In this group, the specific intent of education is reassurance delivered as soon as possible but without the urgency associated with the higher risk group. Information should be provided in the context of the general education provided to all individuals with epilepsy. The clinician should be aware of the potential of the "not asked question." Just because a patient or caregiver does not specifically ask about SUDEP does not mean they do not have concerns or anxiety. The same principles of when, what, and how can be applied to the lower-risk population.

SUMMARY

Patient education in epilepsy is one part of quality epilepsy care and is an evolving and growing field of its own. Although there may be many barriers to providing appropriate and effective education in some settings, there are even more compelling reasons to educate patients and their families. Health outcomes, patient satisfaction, safety, patient/provider communication, and quality of life may all be affected by what people are taught (or not taught), what they understand, and how they use this information to make decisions and manage their health. Data regarding learning needs and interventions to address medication adherence and SUDEP education can be used to guide clinicians in health care or community settings. Ideally, clinicians can enhance their individual educational efforts by encouraging the use of credible community and online information and resources to improve access to epilepsy information and support.

REFERENCES

1. Dilorio C. Epilepsy self-management. Handbook of health behavior research II: provider determinants. New York: Plenum Press; 1997. p. 213–30.

2. Shegog R, Bamps YA, Patel A, et al. Managing Epilepsy Well: emerging e-tools for epilepsy self-management. Epilepsy Behav 2013;29:133–40.

3. Epilepsy Foundation of America. Living well with epilepsy II: report of the 2003 National Conference on Public Health and Epilepsy. Priorities for a public health agenda on epilepsy. Landover (MD): 2003.

4. IOM (Institute of Medicine). Epilepsy across the spectrum: promoting health and understanding. Washington, DC: The National Academies Press; 2012.

5. Dilorio C, Shafer PO, Letz R, et al. Project Ease: a study to test a psychosocial model of epilepsy medication management. Epilepsy Behav 2004;5(6):926–36.

6. Buelow JM, Johnson J. Self-management of epilepsy: A review of the concept and its outcomes. Disease Management and Health Outcomes 2000;8(6): 327–36.

7. Buelow JM. Epilepsy management and issues and techniques. Journal of Neuroscience Nursing 2001;33(5):260–9.

8. Shafer PO, DiIorio C. Managing life issues in epilepsy. Continuum: Lifelong Learning in Neurology - Epilepsy 2004;10(4):138–56.

9. Edward K, Cook M, Giandinoto J. An integrative review of the benefits of self-management interventions for adults with epilepsy. Epilepsy Behav 2015;45: 195–204.

10. Shafer PO. Behavioral therapies in the treatment of adults with epilepsy. In: Schachter SC, editor. Evidence-based management of epilepsy. Harley (Australia): TFM Limited; 2011. p. 143–62.

11. Cochrane J. Patient education: Lessons from epilepsy. Patient Education and Counseling 1995;26(1-3):25–31.

12. Begley C, Shegog R, Harding A, et al. Lingitudinal feasibility of MINDSET: a clinic decision aid for epilepsy self-management. Epilepsy Behav 2015;44:143–50.

13. Faught RE, Duh MS, Weiner JR, et al. Nonadherence to antiepileptic drugs and increased mortality: findings from the RANSOM study. Neurology 2008;71(20): 1572–8.

14. Faught RE, Weiner JR, Guerin A, et al. Impact of nonadherence to antiepileptic drugs on health care utilization and costs: findings from the RANSOM study. Epilepsia 2009;50(3):501–9.

15. Davis KL, Candrilli SD, Edin HM. Prevalence and cost of nonadherence with antiepileptic drugs in an adult managed care population. Epilepsia 2008;49(3): 446–54.

16. Cramer JA, Glassman M, Rienzi V. The relationship between poor medication compliance and seizures. Epilepsy Behav 2002;3(4):338–42.

17. Liu L, Yiu CH, Yen DJ, et al. Medication education for patients with epilepsy in Taiwan. Seizure 2003;12(7):473–7.

18. Tang F, Zhu G, Jiao Z, et al. The effects of medication education and behavioral intervention on Chinese patients with epilepsy. Epilepsy Behav 2014;37:157–64.

19. Helgeson DC, Mittan R, Tan SY, et al. Sepulveda epilepsy education: the efficacy of a psychoeducational treatment program in treating medical and psychosocial aspects of epilepsy. Epilepsia 1990;31:75–82.

20. Ibinda F, Mbuba CK, Kariuki SM, et al. Evaluation of Kilifi epilepsy education programme: a randomized controlled trial. Epilepsia 2014;55(2):344–52.

21. Dash D, Sebastian TM, Aggarwal M, et al. Impact of health education on drug adherence and self-care in people with epilepsy with low education. Epilepsy Behav 2015;44:213–7.

22. Pakpour AH, Gholami M, Esmaeili R, et al. A randomized controlled multimodal behavioral intervention for improving antiepileptic drug adherence. Epilepsy Behav 2015;52:133–42.

23. Plumpton CO, Brown I, Reuber M, et al. Economic evaluation of a behavior-modifying intervention to enhance antiepileptic drug adherence. Epilepsy Behav 2015;45:180–6.

24. Walker ER, Bamps Y, Burdett A, et al. Social support for self-management behaviors among people with epilepsy: a content analysis of the WebEase program. Epilepsy Behav 2012;23(3):285–90.

25. DiIorio C, Bamps Y, Walker ER, et al. Results of a research study evaluating Web-Ease, an online epilepsy self-management program. Epilepsy Behav 2011;22(3): 469–74.

26. Annegers JF. United States perspective on definitions and classifications. Epilepsia 1997;38(11 Suppl):S9–12.

27. Nashef L. Sudden unexpected death in epilepsy: terminology and definitions. Epilepsia 1997;38(11 Suppl):S6–8.

28. Nashef L, So EL, Ryvlin P, et al. Unifying the definitions of sudden unexpected death in epilepsy. Epilepsia 2012;53(2):227–33.

29. Beran RG. SUDEP–to discuss or not discuss: that is the question. Lancet Neurol 2006;5(6):464–5.

30. Morton B, Richardson A, Duncan S. Sudden unexpected death in epilepsy (SUDEP): don't ask, don't tell? J Neurol Neurosurg Psychiatry 2006;77(2):199–202.

31. Hirsch LJ, Donner EJ, So EL, et al. Abbreviated report of the NIH/NINDS workshop on sudden unexpected death in epilepsy. Neurology 2011;76(22):1932–8.

32. Lewis S, Higgins S, Goodwin M. Informing patients about sudden unexpected death in epilepsy: a survey of specialist nurses. Br J Neurosci Nurs 2008;4:5.

33. Gayatri NA, Morrall MC, Jain V, et al. Parental and physician beliefs regarding the provision and content of written sudden unexpected death in epilepsy (SUDEP) information. Epilepsia 2010;51(5):777–82.

34. Vegni E, Leone D, Canevini MP, et al. Sudden unexpected death in epilepsy (SUDEP): a pilot study on truth telling among Italian epileptologists. Neurol Sci 2011; 32(2):331–5.

35. Friedman DE, Donner J, Stephens D, et al. Sudden unexpected death in epilepsy: knowledge and experience among U.S. and Canadian neurologists. Epilepsy Behav 2014;35:13–8.

36. Ramachandrannair R, Jack SM, Meaney BF, et al. SUDEP: what do parents want to know? Epilepsy Behav 2013;29(3):560–4.

37. Xu Z, Ayyappan S, Seneviratne U. Sudden unexpected death in epilepsy (SUDEP): what do patients think? Epilepsy Behav 2015;42:29–34.

38. Tonberg A, Harden J, McLellan A, et al. A qualitative study of the reactions of young adults with epilepsy to SUDEP disclosure, perceptions of risks, views on the timing of disclosure, and behavioral change. Epilepsy Behav 2015;42: 98–106.

39. Devinsky O. Sudden, unexpected death in epilepsy. N Engl J Med 2011;365(19): 1801–11.

40. Hemery C, Ryvlin P, Rheims S. Prevention of generalized tonic-clonic seizures in refractory focal epilepsy: a meta-analysis. Epilepsia 2014;55(11):1789–99.

41. Surges R, Thijs RD, Tan HL, et al. Sudden unexpected death in epilepsy: risk factors and potential pathomechanisms. Nat Rev Neurol 2009;5(9):492–504.

42. Tomson T, Nashef L, Ryvlin P. Sudden unexpected death in epilepsy: current knowledge and future directions. Lancet Neurol 2008;7(11):1021–31.

43. Walczak TS, Leppik IE, D'Amelio M, et al. Incidence and risk factors in sudden unexpected death in epilepsy: a prospective cohort study. Neurology 2001; 56(4):519–25.

Index

Note: Page numbers of article titles are in **boldface** type.

A

AAN. *See* American Academy of Neurology (AAN)
Acetazolamide
    for catamenial epilepsy, 414
AEDs. *See* Antiepileptic drugs (AEDs)
American Academy of Neurology (AAN)
    quality measure sets of
        2009 quality measure set, 320–321
        2014 quality measure set, 322
Antiepileptic drugs (AEDs)
    adherence to
        patient education related to, 449–451
            online educational self-management program, 450–451
            printed drug information, 449–450
            seizure diaries and reminders, 451
            self-administered questionnaire, 450
            structured educational programs, 450
    in epilepsy management, **363–381**
        characteristics of, 365–368
        discontinuing of, 374–377
        efficacy-related issues with
            changing drugs due to, 372–373
        in the elderly, 374
        future directions in, 377–378
        initiation of, 364–369
        tolerability-related issues with
            changing drugs due to, 374
        treatment effects of
            in new-onset epilepsy, 369–372
    QOL in epilepsy related to effects of, 397
    in women with epilepsy
        during pregnancy
            birth outcomes, 419
            cognitive and behavioral teratogenesis, 418–419
            congenital malformations risk associated with, 416
            metabolism and management of, 419–420
            monotherapies, 416–417
            polytherapy, 417–418
        reproductive hormone effects of, 415
        reproductive hormones effects on, 415

Neurol Clin 34 (2016) 457–465
http://dx.doi.org/10.1016/S0733-8619(16)00011-6
0733-8619/16/$ – see front matter © 2016 Elsevier Inc. All rights reserved.

neurologic.theclinics.com

Anxiety
    in epilepsy
        defined, 352–354
        epidemiology of, 352–354
        impact of, 352–354
        introduction, 351–352
        measuring of, 354
        screening for, **351–361**
            considerations/knowledge gaps in, 359
            described, 354–355
            self-report methods in, 356–358
            semi-structured interviews in, 356
            structured interviews in, 355–356
            tools in, 355–359

B

Breastfeeding
    in women with epilepsy, 420

C

Catamenial epilepsy, 412–414
    described, 412
    diagnosis of
        criteria for, 413
    menstrual cycle in, 412–413
    treatment of
        acetazolamide in, 414
        progesterone therapy in, 413–414
Chalfont Seizure Severity Scale, 385
Children
    epilepsy in
        guidelines and quality standards in care of, **327–337** (*See also* Clinical
            practice guidelines (CPGs), for children with epilepsy)
            appraisal of, 334
            audit and benchmarking, 335
            clinical networks, 335
            CPGs, 329–332 (*See also* Clinical practice guidelines (CPGs), for
                children with epilepsy)
            definitions of guidelines, 328–329
            dissemination, 334
            education and training, 335
            evidence-based guidelines, 332
            guideline development in United Kingdom, 327–328
            implementation of, 333–335
            qualitative literature, 332–333
            quality standards, 335
            workforce planning, 335
CIDI. *See* Composite International Diagnostic Interview (CIDI)

Clinical practice guidelines (CPGs)
    for adults with epilepsy, **313–319**
        clinically focused guidelines, 314–315
        comprehensive guidelines, 315–319
    for children with epilepsy
        components of, 329–332
            clarity of presentation, applicability, and editorial independence, 331–332
            evidence and recommendations, 331
            guideline development, 331
            scope, 329
            stakeholder involvement, 329
        qualitative literature in, 332–333
Cognition
    QOL in epilepsy related to, 397
Cognitive assessment
    in initial evaluation of patients with suspected epilepsy, 347
Composite International Diagnostic Interview (CIDI)
    in screening for depression and anxiety in epilepsy, 355
Contraception
    in women with epilepsy, 415–416
CPGs. *See* Clinical practice guidelines (CPGs)

D

Depression
    in epilepsy
        defined, 352–354
        epidemiology of, 352–354
        impact of, 352–354
        introduction, 351–352
        measuring of, 354
        screening for, **351–361**
            considerations/knowledge gaps in, 359
            described, 354–355
            self-report methods in, 356–358
            semi-structured interviews in, 356
            structured interviews in, 355–356
            tools in, 355–359
Diagnostic and Statistical Manual of Mental Disorders (DSM)
    SCID of
        in screening for depression and anxiety in epilepsy, 356
Diary(s)
    seizure, 385–386
        in AEDs adherence, 451
Driver(s) with epilepsy
    reporting of, 431
Driving
    epilepsy and, **427–433**
        background on, 428–429
        commercial driving rules, 433

Driving (*continued*)
    driving standards, regulations, and practices, 429–430
    issues related to, 431–433
    reporting drivers with epilepsy, 431
Drug(s)
    in epilepsy management, **363–381** (*See also specific types and* Antiepileptic
        drugs (AEDs), in epilepsy management)
DSM. *See Diagnostic and Statistical Manual of Mental Disorders* (DSM)

E

EEG. *See* Electroencephalography (EEG)
Elderly
    AEDs in, 374
Electrodermal response
    to seizures, 387–388
Electroencephalography (EEG)
    in seizure monitoring, 388–391
Employment
    epilepsy and, **433–439**
        introduction, 433–435
        issues related to, 437
        military service–related, 437–439
        safety and prevention issues, 436
        standards for, 435–436
Epilepsy. *See also* Seizure(s)
    catamenial, 412–414 (*See also* Catamenial epilepsy)
    defined, 340
    depression and anxiety in
        screening for, **351–361** (*See also* Anxiety, in epilepsy; Depression, in epilepsy)
    described, 363, 427–428
    diagnosis of, 341
    driving and, **427–433** (*See also* Driving, epilepsy and)
    employment and, **433–439** (*See also* Employment, epilepsy and)
    federal disability benefits and, 437–439
    guidelines and quality standards for adults with, **313–325** (*See also* Clinical practice
        guidelines (CPGs), for adults with epilepsy; Quality indicators and measures, for
        adults with epilepsy)
    new-onset
        AEDs effects on, 369–372
    patient education related to, **443–456** (*See also* Patient education, epilepsy-related)
    QOL in people with, **395–410** (*See also* Quality of life (QOL), in people with epilepsy)
    self-management in, 444–451 (*See also* Self-management, in epilepsy)
    suspected
        after single seizure, 341
        initial evaluation of patient with, **339–350**
            determination of type of seizure and epilepsy, 345–346
            early referral to specialized centers in, 347–348
            guiding therapy and prognosis in, 346
            initial assessment in, 345

introduction, 339–340
    psychological and cognitive assessment in, 347
    role of, 342–345
treatment of
    AEDs in, **363–381** (*See also* Antiepileptic drugs (AEDs))
    in women
        issues related to, **411–425** (*See also* Women, epilepsy in)
Epilepsy syndromes
    classification of, 341–342
Evidence-based guidelines
    for children with epilepsy
        weaknesses of, 332

F

Federal disability benefits
    epilepsy and, 437–439
Folic acid
    in women with epilepsy during pregnancy, 419

G

GAD-7. *See* Generalized Anxiety Disorder-7 (GAD-7)
Generalized Anxiety Disorder-7 (GAD-7)
    in screening for depression and anxiety in epilepsy, 358

H

HADS. *See* Hospital Anxiety and Depression Scale (HADS)
Hospital Anxiety and Depression Scale (HADS)
    in screening for depression and anxiety in epilepsy, 358

I

Interview(s)
    in screening for depression and anxiety in epilepsy, 355–356

L

Liverpool Seizure Severity Scale, 384

M

Major depressive episode (MDE)
    defined, 352
MDE. *See* Major depressive episode (MDE)
Menopause
    in women with epilepsy, 420–421
Menstrual cycle
    in catamenial epilepsy, 412–413

Migraine
    QOL in epilepsy related to, 397–398
Military service
    epilepsy and, 437–439
MINI. See Mini-International Neuropsychiatric Interview (MINI)
Mini-International Neuropsychiatric Interview (MINI)
    in screening for depression and anxiety in epilepsy, 355–356

N

NDDI-E. See Neurologic Disorders Depression Inventory for Epilepsy (NDDI-E)
Neurocognitive assessment
    in initial evaluation of patients with suspected epilepsy, 347
Neurologic Disorders Depression Inventory for Epilepsy (NDDI-E)
    in screening for depression and anxiety in epilepsy, 357
Neurosteroid(s)
    in women with epilepsy, 411–412
New-onset epilepsy
    AEDs effects on, 369–372

P

Patient education
    epilepsy-related, **443–456**
        components of, 444–445
        goals of, 444
        introduction, 443–444
        learning needs in, 445–446
        medication adherence in, 449–451
        outcomes of, 445
        setting priorities in, 447
        timing of, 447–449
Patient Health Questionnaire (PHQ-9)
    in screening for depression and anxiety in epilepsy, 356–357
Personal Impact of Epilepsy Scale (PIES), 385
PHQ-9. See Patient Health Questionnaire (PHQ-9)
PIES. See Personal Impact of Epilepsy Scale (PIES)
Pregnancy
    in women with epilepsy, 416–420
        AED birth outcome–related effects, 419
        AED metabolism and management during, 419–420
        AED monotherapies effects on, 416–417
        AED polytherapy effects on, 417–418
        congenital malformations risk with AEDs use, 416
        folic acid use during, 419
Progesterone therapy
    for catamenial epilepsy, 413–414
Psychiatric comorbidities
    QOL in epilepsy related to, 396–397
Psychological evaluation
    in initial evaluation of patients with suspected epilepsy, 347

Q

QOL. *See* Quality of life (QOL)
Quality indicators and measures
    for adults with epilepsy, 314, **319–322**
        AAN 2009 quality measure sets in, 320–321
        described, 319
        history of, 320
        implementation of, 322
Quality of life (QOL)
    in people with epilepsy, **395–410**
        assessment of, 398–399
        determinants of, 396–398
            AED effects, 397
            cognition, 397
            migraine, 397–398
            psychiatric comorbidities, 396–397
            seizures, 396
            sleep, 397
            social impairments, 398
        improving
            self-management strategies in, 406–407
        introduction, 395
        medication effects on
            assessment of, 399–406

R

Reproductive dysfunction
    in women with epilepsy, 414
Reproductive hormones
    AEDs effects on
        in women with epilepsy, 415
    effects on AEDs
        in women with epilepsy, 415

S

SCID for *DSM. See* Structured Clinical Interview (SCID) for *DSM*
Seizure(s), **383–394**. *See also* Epilepsy
    classification of, 341–342
    diaries of, 385–386
        in AEDs adherence, 451
    EEG monitoring of, 388–391
    electrodermal response to, 387–388
    introduction, 383
    QOL in epilepsy related to, 396
    severity of
        scales measuring, 384–385
    shake detectors for, 386–387
    single

Seizure(s) (*continued*)
        epilepsy risk factors after, 341
    tracking of
        methods for, 384
Seizure severity scales, 384–385
Self-management
    in epilepsy
        goals of, 444
        learning needs in, 445–446
        medication adherence in, 449–451
        outcomes of, 445
        setting priorities in, 447
Self-report methods
    in screening for depression and anxiety in epilepsy, 356–358
        GAD-7, 358
        HADS, 358
        NDDI-E, 357
        PHQ-9, 356–357
Semi-structured interviews
    in screening for depression and anxiety in epilepsy, 356
Sex steroid hormone axis
    in women with epilepsy, 412
Sexual dysfunction
    in women with epilepsy, 414
Shake detectors
    seizure-related, 386–387
Sleep
    QOL in epilepsy related to, 397
Social impairments
    QOL in epilepsy related to, 398
Structured Clinical Interview (SCID) for *DSM*
    in screening for depression and anxiety in epilepsy, 356
Structured interviews
    in screening for depression and anxiety in epilepsy, 355–356
Sudden unexpected death in epilepsy (SUDEP)
    patient education related to, 451–454
        discussing, 451–452
        general practices for, 453–454
        patient and family preferences for, 453
        provider preferences for, 452
SUDEP (sudden unexpected death in epilepsy)
    patient education related to, 451–454 (*See also* Sudden unexpected
        death in epilepsy (SUDEP))

    W

Women
    epilepsy in
        introduction, 411
        issues related to, **411–425**
            AED effects on reproductive hormones, 415

breastfeeding, 420
catamenial epilepsy, 412–414 (*See also* Catamenial epilepsy)
contraception, 415–416
menopause, 420–421
neurosteroids, 411–412
pregnancy-related, 416–420 (*See also* Pregnancy, in women with epilepsy)
reproductive and sexual dysfunction, 414
reproductive hormones effects on AEDs, 415
sex steroid hormone axis, 412

Moving?

Make sure your subscription moves with you!

To notify us of your new address, find your **Clinics Account Number** (located on your mailing label above your name), and contact customer service at:

Email: journalscustomerservice-usa@elsevier.com

800-654-2452 (subscribers in the U.S. & Canada)
314-447-8871 (subscribers outside of the U.S. & Canada)

Fax number: 314-447-8029

Elsevier Health Sciences Division
Subscription Customer Service
3251 Riverport Lane
Maryland Heights, MO 63043